BUILT

FOR

SEX

**THE COMPLETE FITNESS AND NUTRITION
PROGRAM FOR MAXIMUM PERFORMANCE**

SCOTT HAYS

RODALE

NOTICE
This book is intended as a reference volume only, not as a medical manual.
The information given here is designed to help you make informed decisions
about your health. It is not intended as a substitute for any treatment that may
have been prescribed by your doctor. If you suspect that you have a medical
problem, we urge you to seek competent medical help.

Mention of specific companies, organizations, or authorities in this book does
not imply endorsement by the publisher, nor does mention of specific companies,
organizations, or authorities imply that they endorse this book.

Internet addresses and telephone numbers given in this book
were accurate at the time it went to press.

SEX AND VALUES AT RODALE
We believe that an active and healthy sex life, based on mutual consent and respect
between partners, is an important component of physical and mental well-being.
We also respect that sex is a private matter and that each person has a different
opinion of what sexual practices or levels of discourse are appropriate. Rodale is
committed to offering responsible, practical advice about sexual matters, supported
by accredited professionals and legitimate scientific research. Our goal—for sex
and all other topics—is to publish information that empowers people's lives.

Rodale books may be purchased for business or promotional use
or for special sales. For information, please write to:
Special Markets Department, Rodale, Inc.,
733 Third Avenue, New York, NY 10017

Printed in the United States of America
Rodale Inc. makes every effort to use acid-free ∞, recycled paper ♺.

Book Design by Susan P. Eugster

Illustrations by Craig L. Kiefer & Kimberly A. Martens
Photographs by Mitch Mandel

Library of Congress Cataloging-in-Publication Data

Hays, Scott Robert, date.
    Built for sex : the complete fitness and nutrition program for maximum
performance / Scott Hays.
        p.   cm.
    Includes index.
    ISBN 13 978–1–57954–978–7 paperback
    ISBN 10 1–57954–978–0 paperback
    1. Men—Health and hygiene. 2. Sex instruction for men.
    3. Men—Sexual behavior. 4. Sex—Health aspects. 5. Sex. I. Title.
RA777.8.H39   2006
613'.04234—dc22   2004016919

Distributed to the trade by Holtzbrinck Publishers

2 4 6 8 10 9 7 5 3 1   paperback

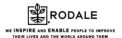

WE INSPIRE AND ENABLE PEOPLE TO IMPROVE
THEIR LIVES AND THE WORLD AROUND THEM

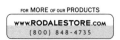

FOR MORE OF OUR PRODUCTS
WWW.RODALESTORE.COM
(800) 848-4735

CONTENTS

ACKNOWLEDGMENTS

THIS BOOK COULD NOT HAVE BEEN WRITTEN WITHOUT THE SUPPORT AND ENCOURAGEMENT OF SEVERAL INDIVIDUALS IN MY LIFE. I wish to extend my deepest appreciation to all of them, especially my girlfriend of nearly a decade, Marty, who's the only one who can truly appreciate what it's like to live with someone like me.

For his insights into strength conditioning and sex, I'd like to thank personal fitness trainer and consultant Don Alessi of AlessiFit.com. For the eating plan and nutritional analysis, special thanks to Kathleen Hanuschak, R.D. For their research and editing skills, I'd like to thank Adrienne Kreger-May and Leah Flickinger at Rodale, and Kevin Jeys, Taran March, and Nan Kappeler. For his research into how many calories it takes to keep a body fit, I'd like to thank Lou Schuler, author of *The Testosterone Advantage Plan*.

THE BLOODFLOW FACTOR

IF YOU'VE EVER SPENT ANY TIME AT A GYM, YOU'VE SEEN HIM. PERHAPS (WE HOPE NOT) YOU EVEN ARE HIM.

We're talking about the guy who goes to the gym, suits up, and then goes around making chin music to everyone else in the place. Sometimes he'll do a couple of stretches or a few half-hearted lifts or maybe take a desultory stroll on the treadmill. But most of the time, he beats his gums. And most important of all, he never—re-peat, never—breaks a sweat.

Now do you know who we're talking about? It's not just that he's not serious. It's the way he always gets in your way. Like when you're trying to work through a few sets of weights, and he's using the leg-press machine as a La-Z-Boy.

We're being pretty hard on the poor guy, but only to emphasize that motivation is the key to having great sex. Every one of us, including this dope at the gym, is a collection of habits. Who we are, how we look, and how we perform in bed are in many ways products of that collection. If, for example, your particular collection of habits includes frequent trips to the kitchen between innings on TV, it's a pretty safe bet that you aren't in the best shape of your life. If you always have sex in the same position or come after a certain length of time, chances are you're going to keep doing it unless you put out the energy to change. And that takes work, commitment, and a *desire* to change.

Unless you're willing to devote enormous time and effort to working out, you are probably never going to have abs like the washboards you see on male fashion models. Hard work and dedication will get you fit—fitter than you've ever been in your life. But you won't get that "shredded" look unless nature designed you that way in the first place.

The same is true of penis size, or how often you can make love in a night, or how often you even want to make love. Your lifestyle—how well you eat, how much you exercise, and so on—can certainly prime the pump and make you feel sexy. It can give you the stamina you need for good sex. It can make you sexy to others. But it won't turn you into some kind of Hollywood sex-puppy. That's not realistic. Nor, for that matter, is it necessary.

A REAL PLAN FOR REAL MEN

When we were researching this book, we talked to a lot of you guys. As you'll see in later chapters, you had a lot of enlightening stuff to say. For starters, you told us you wanted better sex but didn't want to work too hard. The good news is, you don't really have to. Yes, changing your lifestyle and paying attention to the little things takes work, but you're already closer than you think to being attractive to women and having a steamy sex life. How do we know this? When researching the book, we also asked the people who care about how you look and what you do in bed—women. You'll find their voices throughout this book, too. They told us, again and again, that they don't want a man who looks like he lives in a gym. That ripped male physique? It leaves them cold. What they really want is a man who cares enough about himself to stay fit, who can find his way around the kitchen without getting lost, who knows the differences between acrobatic, show-off sex and truly intimate (and hot) encounters.

Six-pack abs and bulging biceps? *"No way!"* a 25-year-old graduate student in New York City told us. *"A guy who's in that kind of shape spends way too much time in front of the mirror. I care about a man's inner beauty, his charm and charisma. That's what makes him sexy."*

The *Built for Sex* plan is based on one simple premise: Every man, whatever his age, diet, or level of fitness, can improve his sex life by making *minimal* changes in his life. Take a moment to let that sink in. You don't need to work out day and night. You don't need to become a vegetarian. You don't have to spend a month's salary on how-to sex books (though the photographs are certainly worth a look). All you have to do is find in yourself the motivation to *tweak* your life rather than turn it upside down.

Here's an example. Doctors who specialize in male sexual problems see a lot of guys who don't get as hard as they'd like. Sure, you can shell out about $10 for a single dose of Viagra or spend a year on a psychologist's couch. But first, try two things and two things only: Improve your diet, and exercise most days of the week. The research is very clear that men who do these two things have better bloodflow, more energy, and enhanced libido. That's one heck of a payoff for two easy changes. Add a couple more tweaks, such as exercises to boost stamina or techniques to intensify orgasms, and the payoff will be even better.

Here are the nuts and bolts of the *Built for Sex* plan. We cover each of these topics in a *lot* more detail later on, but these are the basics.

STEP 1: HONE YOUR TECHNIQUE

We're all creatures of habit. If you've been with the same partner for a long time, you've probably settled into a comfortable routine: A little kissing, a little foreplay, the same sexual positions. There's certainly nothing wrong with familiarity. Couples usually make love in the same ways because they like the way they feel. On the other hand, sexual ruts can be a real stumbling block if they arise more from routine than from real desire.

A lot of the how-to sex guides seem to assume that every man has joints of rubber and the strength to stand on his head, caress his partner, and have mind-blowing sex all at the same time. In real life, though, few of us have the energy (or the interest) to turn the pursuit of pleasure into bedroom gymnastics. What you can, and should, do is occasionally shake things up in bed. Novelty is a tremendous aphrodisiac.

TALK OFTEN, IN AND OUT OF BED. It's hard for men as well as women to say clearly what they want in bed, especially if the things they want seem a little out there. Hey, your partner isn't a mind reader. Sure, a well-timed moan or a little bit of hand pressure speaks volumes about what's working. But you'll never know exactly what your partner wants you to do, or what you want her to do to you, unless you speak up.

Do you want more strength and pressure when she plays with you? Tell her. Do you prefer aggressive oral sex or light touches and teasing? Say so. Do you have fantasies about being totally passive—or, conversely, taking total control? Talk about it. Each man and woman has different desires, different likes and dislikes. Don't leave it all to chance.

TRY ALL-DAY FOREPLAY. Sex doesn't begin when you turn out the lights. Couples who report being happiest with their sex lives invariably spend a lot of time flirting, teasing, and playing. They don't wait until they're undressed. They trade sexy phone calls, full-body hugs in the hall, quick kisses that are more than a peck on the lips. Hot sex requires more than 0-to-60 intensity. You have to keep the embers glowing.

PLAY WITH POSITIONS. Even if you have a couple of favorites, take the initiative to do something new. Sex from behind instead of man on top. Interrupt intercourse to have oral sex rather than using your mouth only during foreplay. Try it standing, sitting, lying down. The great thing about sex is that there isn't a statute of limitations on play; you can experiment as often and in as many different ways as you like. As with anything else, it doesn't always work. You might find yourself doing more laughing than anything else. That's okay. That's great, actually. Intimacy means trusting each other enough to try just about anything. Don't worry about where you're going. Enjoy the journey.

STEP 2: MAXIMIZE CONTROL

Maybe you're always hard when you want to be. Maybe you always come right when you want to. Maybe you always have the stamina to please your partner the way she wants to be pleased. Maybe you walk on water and can levitate a bottle of Bud from the refrigerator to the living room couch.

Unless you're a magician (or less than honest), sexual embarrassment is a fact of life. *Every* man has occasions when his body won't perform, when the heat of the moment gets doused with the cold water of a flagging erection or too-quick ejaculation. These and other sexual letdowns have little to do with your genetic makeup. Even when they're caused by physical problems—for example, buildups of cholesterol that inhibit bloodflow to the penis—they can almost always be minimized with a combination of exercise and lifestyle changes.

Did you know, for example, that you can dramatically improve your "holding" power with a series of exercises that takes just a couple of minutes a day? It's true. Specialists in sexual dysfunction clinics report that the vast majority of men who suffer from premature ejaculation can gain significant control by combining Kegel exercises with "squeeze" techniques that slow the rush to orgasm.

Want more motivation? Consider this: Men who practice these techniques—even men who already have good ejaculatory control—frequently report stronger and more intense orgasms. Along the way, some even develop the ability to have multiple orgasms.

STEP 3: EXERCISE FOR BETTER SEX

Stretching, strength training, and cardiovascular workouts are the guts of the *Built for Sex* plan. Exercise increases the flow of energizing endorphins and adrenaline, body chemicals that make you feel strong, sexy, and confident. Guys who work out tend to have higher levels of testosterone, the male hormone you need for arousal as well as performance. Researchers at Cologne University Medical Centre in Germany even found that men who exercise have substantial increases of bloodflow to the penis—bloodflow that you need for erections.

We're not talking hard-core athletics. Men who work out *moderately* have increased sex drive and more predictable erections. In a landmark study, 78 sedentary, middle-age men did nothing more than aerobics four times a week. When researchers talked to them 9 months later, they learned that their frequency of sex had increased by nearly a third, and the frequency of orgasms had increased 26 percent.

And there are other exercise payoffs.

INCREASED CONFIDENCE. Men who exercise feel stronger and more energetic. They have more physical and mental confidence. They feel good in their own skins, and this goes a long way in the sexual realm.

MORE ENERGY. Even moderate levels of exercise—lifting a couple of times a week, for example, or taking daily walks—can stave off sex-killing fatigue. As a 54-year-old technical writer from Phoenix told us, *"I was sucking down pastries, chips, and sodas, and I was tired all the time. About a year ago, I made up my mind to get back to exercising, eating the right foods, and walking at lunch. I think my hormone levels must be up, because I want sex all the time."*

LOOKING BETTER. Lift weights a couple of times a week for a few months, and you're going to see the difference. You'll feel better when you look in the mirror. Your partner will enjoy looking at you. Now that's sexy.

BETTER SEX. The more you exercise, the more blood arrives in the penis. More blood means better erections. You'll be able to go longer without fatigue. And you'll *want* sex more than you did before.

You'll also be stronger and more limber—qualities you'll need if you even hope to try some of the more creative positions out there. Whether you want to get creative or stick with the tried and true, one simple exercise can kick it up a notch. Look at the "Position of Strength" section in chapter 8 for the specific exercise that strengthens the muscles you use for your favorite positions.

LESS STRESS. It's probably the main factor in low libido as well as erection problems. In fact, men who are stressed all the time find it almost impossible to have good sex because of destructive changes in body chemistry. Research has clearly shown that even lightweight exercise programs, such as occasional lifting, stretching, or aerobics, cause a dramatic drop in stress chemicals and an increase in sexual interest and activities.

BETTER HEALTH. It's hardly a secret that men who exercise are a lot less likely to get diabetes or hypertension, chronic and life-threatening diseases that are among the main causes of sexual problems.

Because exercise is so effective at improving appearance and physical and mental health, we've designed a total fitness plan that includes strength training, stretching, and cardiovascular workouts. You'll get stronger, in and out of bed. You'll have more sexual endurance, and you'll notice improvements in the muscles and joints that you need for good sex. We've even included exercises to improve ejaculatory control and increase the intensity of orgasms.

STEP 4: EAT FOR LOVE

Nutrition is a key component of sexual stamina and love. If you're like most men, you don't give it a lot of thought. Let's face it: The whole idea of nutrition isn't exactly stimulating. It's hard to get excited about something when the payoffs are so far down the road.

We're not about to claim that the usual nutritional advice, like cutting fat from your diet and eating more salad, is likely to hit any of your hot buttons. What we can say, and research backs us up, is that the payoffs can be dramatic. We're not talking all-or-nothing. You don't have to overhaul your diet, throw out the steaks, and empty your cabinets of anything that isn't natural, brown, and tasteless. Relatively small changes can make a huge difference in your health, sexual and otherwise. For example:

GET ALL THE C YOU CAN HANDLE. It's probably the most important nutrient for men. For one thing, it's an antioxidant: It essentially neutralizes harmful molecules (free radicals) that damage cells throughout the body, including cells in the tiny blood vessels in the penis. If you smoke, it's especially important to eat vitamin C–rich foods, such as green vegetables and citrus fruits. It takes about 20 milligrams of vitamin C to squelch the free-radical effects of one cigarette.

Vitamin C does more than improve your overall health; you need it specifically for sex. Men who get as little as 200 milligrams of vitamin C daily have healthier sperm than men who get lower amounts. It also makes it harder for the harmful LDL form of cholesterol to stick to blood vessels and inhibit bloodflow to the penis.

TAKE VITAMIN E SUPPLEMENTS. It's almost always better to get nutrients from foods instead of capsules, but vitamin E is an exception. Even though you can get the Daily Value of 30 IU from cooking oils, nuts, and a few other foods, doctors usually advise men to get up to 400 IU a day. For that, you have to take supplements. It's worth doing because vitamin E can help keep blood flowing through the arteries of the penis. It's especially important to get enough if you have diabetes, one of the leading causes of erection problems.

EAT LESS MEAT AND MORE FISH. Meat, as you know, is loaded with saturated fat, the stuff that's converted in the liver to cholesterol. Fish, as you might not know, is high in omega-3 fatty acids, the types of fat that can improve cholesterol and make it easier for blood to circulate where you need it. Plan on eating fish two or three times a week. Don't fry it, though—it will turn that turbot into a fat torpedo.

GRAZE FROM THE GARDEN. Just about every fruit and vegetable is jammed with antioxidants. Some, like the lycopene in tomatoes, can dramatically reduce your risk of prostate cancer. Broccoli contains sulforaphane, a chemical compound that boosts the body's production of cancer-blocking enzymes. Cabbage, green beans, romaine lettuce, bananas—they all contain substances that can help keep blood flowing and prevent the kinds of cell changes that can lead to cancer and other life-changing health threats.

LOAD UP ON SHELLFISH. With the exception of shrimp, all shellfish are high in zinc, the mineral that's almost custom made for men. It's essential for fertility and prostate health. It helps cuts heal more quickly—important for guys who try to shave and drink coffee at the same time. It also boosts the immune system, which can prevent all sorts of infections, including infections in the prostate gland, from taking hold and dragging you down.

GET YOUR WEIGHT DOWN. If we men ate only when we were hungry, we'd all be as thin as whippets. Unfortunately, though, for us and our bellies, we eat for all sorts of reasons that have nothing to do with hunger. We eat when we're happy, sad, lonely, worried, nervous, tired, and bored. We eat to reward ourselves. We eat because we have a couple of minutes and nothing else to occupy our minds. We eat because it's just about impossible in this country to do anything, including fill your tank with gas, without being surrounded by food.

Those extra pounds do more than send you in search of an upsized wardrobe. They vastly increase your risk of diabetes, which can literally destroy blood vessels and nerves in the penis—bad for that all-important bloodflow. Men who are overweight tend to get tired easily. They don't feel good about themselves when they look in the mirror—or when they realize that their partners aren't looking at them the way they used to.

You know what you have to do. We know what you have to do. The only question is when you'll take the key steps—exercising most days of the week, dropping some of those calories off your plate, and snacking less—that you know will turn things around.

True, most of the women you meet won't care if your physique is less than model-perfect. They're not perfect either and would probably be intimidated by a man who looks too good. That said, women as well as men are most attracted to partners who are at least somewhat fit—and who carry themselves with the kind of confidence that comes from taking good care of yourself.

As a 27-year-old IT technician in Boulder, Colorado, told us, *"I don't mind a man who's a little bit overweight. His belly can even seem a little hot as long as he's comfortable in his own skin. But it's important to me that he respects himself enough to work out and take care of himself generally."*

THE *BUILT FOR SEX* PROMISE

Most of us are unconscious when it comes to our eating, exercise, and sexual habits. We do all sorts of things without really thinking about them. Many of these habits, unfortunately, drag us down rather than build us up. Do you have sex now as much as you did in your randy 20s? Probably not. If you're like most of us, the accrual of responsibilities and stress—job, family, money worries, and fatigue—has gradually eroded your lust for adventure and passion. You haven't given up sex, not by a long shot. You still want to exercise and look good. But do you think about it as much as you used to? Probably not.

You need to take the time to really tune into your life. Get a better sense of how you eat. How you exercise. How you feel when you make love. If you're not entirely satisfied with what you see after a little bit of soul-searching—and it's doubtful that anyone is—it's time to add a couple of new habits and, sure, subtract a couple of the bad ones.

We understand that no man is going to turn his whole life upside down, even for the promise of more and better sex. Well, you don't have to. If you do nothing more than follow the steps in *any one* of the *Built for Sex* programs—technique adjustments, sexual control, strength training, eating right, and more—you're going to notice dramatic changes in how you feel and perform. You'll be a better lover. You'll achieve ejaculatory and erection control that you didn't have before. You'll please your partner more. You'll feel better about your body, your health, and your life.

The biggest challenge, one that's harder than changing your eating habits or contorting your limbs in highly erotic but unfamiliar ways, is to change the way you talk to yourself. Maybe you don't talk aloud, but if you're a man, you do talk to yourself, like cartoon characters who have an angel perched on one shoulder and a devil on the other. Unfortunately, the devil often gives the angel the boot. Not only does he tempt us into sin ("Hey, you're already over-weight, what's another slice of cheesecake?"), he has an even more subtle tool for undercutting your self-confidence. Call it the "if . . . then" way of thinking. "If you can just lose 20 pounds," the devil tells you, "then you'll feel great and have better sex."

That kind of thinking gets you nowhere because the rewards are always delayed. If you're really going to get motivated, you have to learn to appreciate who you are and where you are in your life. Don't start this plan because you're dissatisfied with where you are now. Start it because you know you deserve the best life has to offer, and there's no better time to start than now.

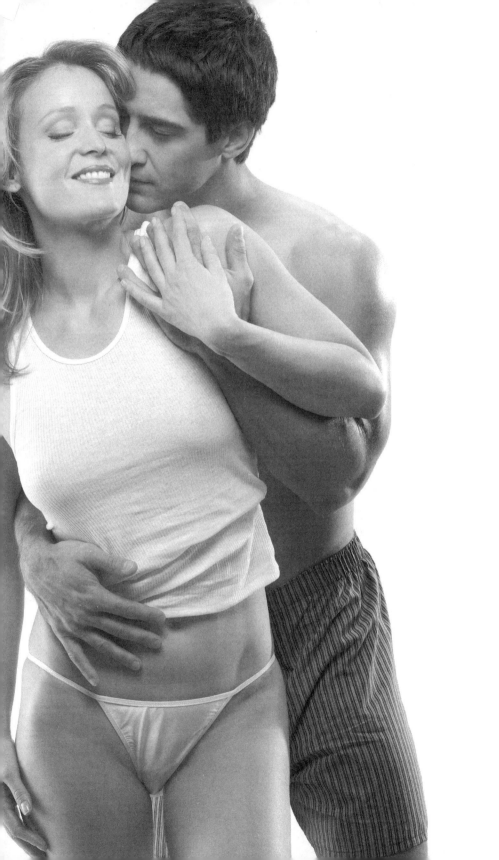

PART 1

HONE YOUR TECHNIQUE

CHAPTER 1

SEX THROUGH THE AGES

BEFORE WE GET INTO THE TECHNICAL NITTY-GRITTY, LET'S FIGURE OUT WHERE YOU ARE ON THE SEXUAL TIMELINE. Why? Because age changes everything, sex included. A 23-year-old cruising a crowded Friday night happy hour isn't thinking about how he'll perform 40 years later, but he should be. The habits we develop early on can have a profound impact on our performance decades down the road.

Even if you've always walked the straight and narrow, your sex life will change as you get older. Some of the changes can only be called improvements; others will have you shaking your head. It's worth taking a quick look at what you're likely to expect—what's normal, what's a problem, and what you can do to stay on top of your game.

SEX AT 19

You've probably heard that men are at their sexual primes at 19. It's not really true, although at that age, the penis gets as hard as it ever will. Erections do get less firm after that, but you're unlikely to notice any significant change in rigidity until you reach your 40s.

In evolutionary terms, this erectile readiness made sense because puberty and reproduction occurred simultaneously. A young man's ability to get hard quickly and repeatedly had more practical utility than it does today.

What exactly does it mean when we say that a man reaches his sexual peak at this age? Basically, it's all about speed. How quickly he gets an erection, how quickly he ejaculates, and how quickly he's ready again. There's certainly something to be said for rapid erections and equally rapid recovery, but it hardly makes much difference, or is even desirable, in a mature relationship.

Men this young are the last ones to seek advice, especially sexual advice, from anyone. That's too bad because this is the age when lifelong sexual habits get started—and when health habits either take root or get thrown in the nearest ditch. If you or someone you know falls in this age group, here are some points to keep in mind.

SLOW DOWN. Too many men, young guys especially, follow the wham-bam style of lovemaking. A 19-year-old is naturally faster on the trigger than a man in his 40s, but he doesn't have to be *that* fast. There are all sorts of exercises that can slow the rush to orgasm. At the very least, men this age should get in the habit of periodically slowing down during intercourse or stopping entirely to change positions or cool down.

SEDUCE. It's true that young men and women, awash in hormones, can go a little sex crazy. It's also true that the role models for too many guys this age are the frat boys in the classic *Animal House*—which is why they spend a lot more time thinking about sex than having sex. Want to woo the women? Take the time to get to know them. Find out about their lives, their interests, their dreams. Apart from the fact that respect is never a bad thing, you'll find that you have a lot more success when you have more than sex in mind.

EAT RIGHT. High cholesterol usually starts to be a health risk for men in their 40s or older, but there's good evidence that the process starts in the teens. Young guys who get all their meals from the drive-thru are laying down arterial deposits that sooner or later will start to jam bloodflow to the penis.

SEX IN THE 20S

For many men, their 20s are the "lost decade," the time when they do things they'll remember (or not) for the rest of their lives. If you can manage to exit the decade without landing in some jail, morgue, or asylum, you'll have plenty of stories to remember fondly when you're old enough to have grandkids.

Most men become sexually active on a consistent basis when they're in their 20s. They have their first serious girlfriends or live-ins. Even if they're single, this is the age when men and women are getting serious about hustling up a mate, or at least some action. It's also the time they begin to define and refine their sexual habits and preferences. They start to discover who they are and what they want as well as how to please and be pleased.

Some men in their mid-20s haven't yet learned to accommodate their partners' needs. A lot of guys fall into this category, at least until they finally get it through their heads that sex isn't all about them.

To get through this decade with a boatload of experience as well as good memories, here's what experts advise.

EXPERIMENT, EXPLORE. Men usually enter their first long-term relationships when they're in their 20s. The relationships are usually disasters. It's difficult to establish and maintain a relationship at any age, but men in their 20s don't yet have a lot of skill at either communication or compromise. To the best of your ability, be open and honest with your partners, especially about sex. Don't pretend to like things you don't. Don't insist that she do things she's not

DOES FINGER SIZE INDICATE PENIS SIZE?

More than a few women (and men) are convinced that men with long fingers have long penises. The same has been said of tall men and men with thick thumbs. Is there any truth to it?

Nope. (Surprise.) Scientists have tried to correlate a number of body attributes with penis size, and it never pans out. Many tall men have small penises. A man with small thumbs could be prodigiously endowed. There's really no way to tell without actually looking if a guy is big, small, or (most likely) absolutely average.

comfortable with. By all means, play. Discover yourself, but be prepared to shift gears quickly when it's obvious things aren't working. Fact: A relationship involves two people. It's not all about you.

TAKE CARE OF YOURSELF. Guys in their 20s tend to lap up liquor all night, then play hard the next day. You can get away with it for a while; your body is resilient at that age. But each bender and bad habit is doing something, even if you can't see it yet. Smoking, heavy drinking, drugs—they take a toll, one that has to be paid sooner or later. Take care of your body now. You'll be grateful you did.

START EXERCISING. You know the ropes: Get out at least three or four times a week. Do some cardio. Lift weights. You start to lose muscle tissue by the time you reach your 30s, so it's good to have some extra in the bank. Besides, the habits you pick up in your 20s are likely to be the ones that follow you around for the next few years (or decades). It's better to make them good ones.

SEX IN THE 30S

As a physical specimen, a man in his 30s should still look and feel pretty good—although this is the time that diseases, even if they haven't hit yet, get their noses under the tent. If you follow the traditional pattern, this is also the decade in which you're most likely to settle into a life of marriage, career, and family. Unfortunately, it's also the decade in which most men start to feel a little uneasy about the directions their lives have taken.

Lifelong monogamy is widespread among neither animals nor humans. In this country, at least, men and women are more likely to practice "serial monogamy." Instead of a single union that lasts until one member of a couple expires, people shift in and out of "committed" couplings, establishing two or more serious relationships during the course of their lives.

The 7-year itch refers to the restlessness many people in long-term relationships eventually experience. You might find that you're no longer in love with the woman you married because you and she have become very different people. Sexual boredom and a drop in libido can take a toll. People have affairs, and more than half of marriages end in divorce, often in the 30s or early 40s.

The 30s, then, is a decade of physical, emotional, and romantic change. Here's how to cope a little better.

REKINDLE THE SPARKS. After the partner-hopping of his 20s, a man in his 30s is usually ready to commit. As the years go by, however, sex tends to get crowded out by bills, diapers, work, and all of the other usual life pressures. Couples who don't make the effort to keep the fire burning soon find themselves bored or resentful. Don't let it happen to you. Set aside time each week to go out to dinner, to a movie—anything to bring back the excitement and intimacy of dating. Relationships need nurturing, or they wither and die.

MAKE THE EXERCISE COMMITMENT. It's tough to find time for regular workouts when you're swamped with work and family obligations. Do it anyway. Your 30s is the time when your less-than-ideal habits from the past start to catch up with you. Exercise will give you the energy to keep going, in bed and out. It will boost your confidence at an age when many men start to feel that youth is gone.

It's also a great way to reduce and manage stress at a time when life pressures are highest.

GET IN THE HABIT OF STRETCHING. Sign up for a yoga class. Take some long walks. Stretch after workouts. Do whatever you have to do to keep your joints and muscles loose and limber. Starting to notice a little twinge in your back or shoulder when you make love? Welcome to the club—you're in your 30s, and those little aches and pains are only going to get worse if you don't get serious about flexing and stretching.

▼

A study that appeared in the _British Medical Journal_ reports that men who have sex at least twice a week have half the death rate of those who have sex once a month. Sex, as defined by the study, included masturbation as well as intercourse.

▲

START LIFTING. Your bone mass increases until about age 35. After that, it holds steady until you're in your 60s, at which point, it starts to decline. You want to build as much bone strength as you can before that happens. That means getting plenty of calcium in your diet and taking up a program of weight-bearing exercise. Lifting weights strengthens bones and keeps them strong, which can dramatically reduce your risk of fractures later on. In the meantime, of course, the added strength will give you extra stamina and enjoyment in the bedroom.

BANISH THAT BELLY. If you're like most men, the 30s is the time when the needle on the scale swings farther to the right than it's ever gone before. If you're getting a little heavier than you'd like, now's the time to take care of it—with diet, exercise, whatever it takes. Remember, the fat cells you create today are with you forever. Whipping yourself into shape now will save you a lot of grief later. In the meantime, staying trim makes looking in the mirror a lot more pleasant.

SHAKE THE SALT. While you're at it, eat a lot more fruits and vegetables and less meat. Blood pressure often starts to rise in a man's

30s. Even though it may take decades before you notice symptoms, all of that turbulence in your arteries can cause long-lasting damage—including damage to the arteries that help you get erections. Your doctor probably checks your blood pressure every time you get a checkup. If he doesn't, insist on it. If you don't catch high blood pressure early, you could find yourself looking at a future of fistfuls of prescription drugs, along with damage to your kidneys, heart, and arteries.

SEX IN THE 40S

On the scale of evolutionary time, it was only yesterday that men even had a chance of living out their 40s, let alone their 50s. This is a frightening time for men. Middle age is close. Your health might not be as good as it used to be. You probably don't get erections as often as you used to. You take longer to get hard, and it takes a lot longer to get hard again.

In fact, men in their 40s are much less likely to get erections from fantasies alone. When they do get erections, they're noticeably less firm than they used to be. The transmission of nerve signals into the penis is less efficient as well.

What can you do? Here are a few places to start.

GET HANDS-ON STIMULATION. Young men get hard at the very thought of sex, but men in their 40s usually need some direct contact. When you're making love, don't hesitate to touch yourself the way you like. Or encourage your partner to use her hands or mouth. Definitely reassure her. She might assume that the time it takes you to get hard is a reflection of your desire (or lack of it) for her. Be honest. Let her know that you're slower than you used to be, but still raring to go.

BE REALISTIC. Young guys can often reload in an hour or two, or often quicker. Men in their 40s may require an entire night—or, commonly, days—before they can have intercourse again. It's a perfectly normal age-related change, so don't get stressed. By all means, have sex as often as you want. Some guys continue to get hard on demand their entire lives. Others don't.

GET SERIOUS ABOUT YOUR DIET. Heart disease is a real risk once you reach your 40s. This is the time to do everything you can to get cholesterol down and keep it down. Most men can do it with diet alone. If you can't, you may need a statin, one of the cholesterol-lowering drugs. Statins are very safe and very effective. And because they help prevent blockages in blood vessels throughout your body, they can help stave off erection problems as well as heart disease and stroke.

WORK OUT MOST DAYS OF THE WEEK. It doesn't matter what you do. Swim if you like. Go for long, fast walks. Lift weights most days. You don't have to be a fanatic. Plan on exercising for at least 30 minutes most days of the week. That's enough to put your cardiovascular system in the safety zone—and to ensure that you maintain the kind of bloodflow that makes erections possible.

According to a recent survey, 98 percent of men would like a larger penis.

KEEP AN EYE ON YOUR WEIGHT. Yep, this is the decade that all of those ice cream cones and T-bones you enjoyed all your life will start stubbornly sticking to your midsection. Men who never had to watch calories before often find in their 40s that their pants are getting a little snug.

Men tend to accumulate fat in the abdomen, the so-called beer belly. The bad news is that this is the kind of weight distribution that dramatically increases your risk of diabetes and heart disease. On the other hand, it's also the kind of fat that's easiest to shed with diet and exercise.

SEX IN THE 50S AND BEYOND

Most of the sexual problems experienced by men in their 50s are due to underlying health problems, such as heart disease and diabetes. At the same time, most men start to have a slight reduction in sex drive—although about two-thirds continue to have sex at least several times a month.

Erection problems get more pronounced during this decade, usually because the connective tissue gets less elastic, and there's often a decline in bloodflow. Orgasms typically get less intense as well. This is also the time when the prostate gland starts to make a nuisance of itself.

A man in his 50s obviously has to do many of the same things as younger men: exercise, eat right, and so on. In addition, he'll need to do a few extra things to keep himself healthy and sexually active.

EAT PLENTY OF TOMATOES. They contain lycopene, a chemical compound that helps protect the prostate gland from cancerous changes. One large study of nearly 48,000 men found that those who ate at least 10 weekly servings of tomatoes (including the tomatoes on pizza and in ketchup) were able to cut their risk of prostate cancer by 45 percent.

▼

The penis usually doubles in size between the ages of 10 and 16. It reaches adult proportions at about age 17.

▲

ASK YOUR DOCTOR ABOUT SAW PAL-METTO. Available in supplement form, it's among the best treatments for benign prostatic hyperplasia, the age-related growth of the prostate gland that can slow or even block the normal flow of urine. There's some evidence that saw palmetto works at least as well as prescription drugs.

GET REGULAR PROSTATE EXAMS. Prostate cancer is silent in the early stages. The only way to catch it at an early, more treatable stage is to get regular checkups that include a digital exam and the PSA, a blood test that checks for cancer markers.

CHECK YOUR MEDS WITH YOUR DOCTOR. Roughly a third of men age 60 and older are unable to get or maintain erections. This is often due to underlying health problems, but it can also be a side effect of common medications, including antidepressants and drugs for high blood pressure. Never assume that it's normal not to get erections; it always means that something's wrong. In some cases, just changing drugs is enough to turn things around.

ASK ABOUT VIAGRA. It's nothing less than a godsend for men with circulatory or other problems that inhibit the flow of blood into the penis. Viagra, along with newer drugs such as Cialis and Levitra, allow more blood to enter the spongy tissue. The vast majority of men who take one of these drugs have better and more frequent erections.

CHAPTER 2

THE THRILL OF SEDUCTION

SEDUCTION RUNS ON THE HIGH-OCTANE FUEL OF UN-CERTAINTY. YOU DON'T KNOW WHAT WILL HAPPEN NEXT. The pleasurable anticipation focuses concentration and heightens all the senses. Things might go well or badly; there's no way to tell. The risk taking of seduction—putting yourself out there in the hopes of taking a relationship to the next level—is inherently thrilling.

This probably explains why laboratory animals, taught to push a button that dispenses the food they love, press it more often when the actual arrival of food is intermittent. It's almost as if they're more excited by the pursuit than by the food itself. When the same animals are permitted to score every time, they soon lose interest and leave the button alone.

Seduction is like that. The element of doubt, those provocative question marks that hover over each glance and casual touch, gives it that erotic, stomach-tingling thrill. At its best, seduction transforms a friendly exchange into one of intimacy and sexual pleasure. It's a skill worth learning. Women *want* to be seduced and tempted.

They want a man who makes them feel special, who cares enough to take his time in the journey from the first interested glance to sensual touches and beyond. What they don't want is a man who takes them for granted, who's so focused on the endgame that he neglects all of the intermediate, and pleasurable, steps.

Consider these words from a 33-year-old marketing coordinator in Morristown, New Jersey. She won't even consider getting into bed with a guy who's obviously looking to score. *"I'm not going to waste my time if he seems like a player—or hand over my number just so I can be frustrated when he doesn't call me."*

Of course, seduction is a bit of an endgame all by itself. It takes time to get there, and you won't even get started unless you pay attention to the 1,001 signals your partner is putting out—and to the messages that you send, deliberately or not. Seduction isn't *all* about sexual mechanics. That comes later. First, you have to get past that initial "hello."

12 STEPS TO SEX APPEAL

The women we surveyed weren't shy about listing the physical qualities they like in a man. They certainly enjoy admiring a man's legs, butt, or biceps. But physical qualities hardly registered on their attraction meters. They were a lot more interested in things like grooming. Good hygiene. Confidence. Sincerity. In short, all of those things that gym rats don't even think about while they're buffing up their six-packs.

Sex appeal is an elusive quality. What one woman finds sexy may cause another to head for the exit. It generally has more to do with inner qualities, such as strength and integrity, than with visible characteristics. A model-handsome man with a great wardrobe and an expensive car will certainly get a woman's attention, but he's unlikely to keep it unless he brings something extra to the table.

And sex appeal isn't just for single men. *"Now that we've been married a few years, my husband doesn't seem to be concerned about looking good for me,"* said a 38-year-old Chicago science teacher. *"And I don't feel that sexual pull as strongly as when we were dating."*

Even though the women we talked to represented just about every age group and profession, they were nearly unanimous about the qualities they found most attractive. All of these qualities are things you already possess—though you might want to take the time to dust them off.

KICK UP YOUR CONFIDENCE. Ask 100 women what they consider sexy, and 99 of them will put confidence first on their list. Don't believe anyone who says you have to be born with it. A lot of what we call confidence is really survival: When you reach a certain age and have experienced more than your share of flaming embarrassments, you tend to learn that anything that doesn't kill you will make you stronger. Knowing the worst that can happen—and knowing that the worst probably isn't too bad—is a superb confidence builder.

More practically, those of us without a lot of natural confidence can learn to fake it. Smiling easily even when you're tense. Standing tall and relaxed when you approach someone at a party. Walking up to a stranger and saying something like, "There's something about you; I didn't want to leave without introducing myself."

Sure, it takes guts to put yourself on the line. You might flub it. You might be left standing with your mouth open and a drink in your hand. But hey, what do you have to lose? Women know that it's hard for men to approach them. No matter how shaky you feel inside, they'll be impressed that you had the *cojones* to take the chance.

STAND UP FOR MANNERS. Some gentlemen might prefer blondes, but rest assured that the women you meet, whatever their hair color, prefer gentlemen. This is no less true in the corner tavern than at the symphony. Guys today have gotten pretty casual. Women accept the reality of modern life—but that doesn't mean they like it. Want to show that you're a cut above the clueless lout in the wife-beater who leers and whistles at every woman who walks by? Take off the baseball cap. Stand up when she approaches the table. Shave now and then. In other words, show her that you won't be a total embarrassment when she introduces you to her friends.

Even if your natural instinct is to pad around in slippers and stained sweats, you'd do well to cultivate some of the vanishing signals of chivalry. Open doors. Call a cab when she leaves the bar. Carry her packages. Offer to bring her a plate at parties. While you're at it, extend the same politeness to waiters, valets, and anyone else you happen to meet. She'll notice and appreciate the gestures. More important, she'll know that she can trust you with her most precious possession—herself. *"Physical attractiveness always helps, but a man with charm wins me over every time,"* said a 28-year-old editorial assistant in Brooklyn.

The first couple to be shown in bed together on prime-time television was Fred and Wilma Flintstone.

LOOK THE PART. Forget the Calvin Klein ads. A 5 o'clock shadow and dirty T-shirt might play into a woman's fantasies of a rugged bad boy, but there's a huge gap between fantasy and real life. Unless you really are a 22-year-old model, don't try to look like one. Women like men who know how to dress. Sure, it's fine to dress down at home, but keep a few pairs of pressed pants around. Tuck in your shirt. Heck, shine your shoes for a change. The "natural" look, taken to extremes, isn't a turn-on for most women. The opposite: It's a sign of immaturity in their eyes. You don't want her to look at you and be reminded of the baggy, pizza-stained garb perpetually hanging off her kid brother.

SHOW SOME SCENTS SENSE. Cologne is risky territory. Women grow up using scents and usually have a pretty good idea of what works. Most men, on the other hand, are amateurs and apt to choose the wrong scents—or worse, douse on too much. Besides, most of the women who answered our survey said that they liked men to smell like men: clean and washed—period.

LEARN TO DANCE. Sorry, there's no getting around it. Women know that they're more likely to find a dancing bear than a dancing man. Refusing to dance won't necessarily ruin your chances, but it sure won't make you stand out from the pack. Most of the dancing people do these days doesn't follow a formula, so just get comfortable on the dance floor and fake it from there. But why not learn a couple of basic ballroom steps so you really stand out? *"I knew I wanted to get to know him better when he dragged me onto the dance floor to do the jitterbug on our first date,"* said a 41-year-old Boston medical researcher of the man she married. No one's expecting you to be Fred Astaire, but a little rhythm and enthusiasm go a long way.

ACT FIT. You'll notice we didn't say "be fit," although it's obviously to your advantage if you are. Physical attributes, as we mentioned, rank pretty low on most women's must-have lists, but physical *confidence* ranks at the top. Women are very tuned in to the way you move and carry yourself. If you slouch, chew your nails, or run your hands compulsively through your hair, you're going to look as insecure as you probably feel. Stand up straight. Walk with purpose. Move as though you know exactly what you want. Sure, it might be a bit of an act, but that's okay. Men who look physically confident get more positive attention than those who don't. Those good vibes that you take in will make you *feel* more confident. That's a cycle you want to cultivate.

STAY REAL. The word *seduction* has a whiff of calculation about it, as though charming and sleeping with a woman is a game

WHAT'S NORMAL?

In the world of sex, not much. Normal implies some sort of ideal, or at least an average, that everyone meshes into. The concept of normal is useful for describing the behavior of large numbers of people, but it totally misses the point when you're talking about you or the guy next to you.

Consider the notion of a normal number of sexual partners. Fifty years ago, the normal man was expected to sleep around a bit. The normal woman, on the other hand, was expected to sleep with one man—her husband—and one man only. Some people undoubtedly fit into these norms, but most didn't. People just lied about it more.

So forget the concept of normal. Let's look instead at what seems to be common—or not.

▶ **Penis size.** Most men measure between 5 and 7 inches. Not sure how you measure up? Drop your pants, and lightly press a ruler against your abdomen alongside your erect penis.

▶ **Orgasmic frequency.** In the 1940s, Dr. Alfred Kinsey interviewed 12,000 men about their sexual habits. The numbers were all over the map. Some men said it was normal for them to come four or five times a day. One gentleman disclosed that he had one orgasm in 30 years. Is there such a thing as normal? Certainly not in this arena.

▶ **Sexual frequency.** About a third of heterosexual American men have sex twice a week or more. Another third has sex a few times a month. The other third has sex, at most, a few times a year.

Recognize yourself in any of these categories? You might and might not because, let's face it, none of us are strictly normal. Which is why we all think, deep in our hearts, that our desires or performance somehow tilt to the abnormal side of things. And *that's* perfectly normal.

to be won. There's a term for guys who work this way. They're known as players, and women can smell them a mile away.

Consider what a 29-year-old graphic designer told us. *"If you attempt to use a pickup line on me, no matter how smooth you think it is, you won't have a chance. Honesty and sincerity win me over all the time."*

All those sexual innuendos and pickup lines you've been practicing since high school? Dump them in the round file. Even if they work, and a woman agrees to go home with you, so what? You'll have a notch on your bedpost and nothing else except regrets when you find yourself, as you invariably will, alone and lonely in the middle of the night.

THROW IN SOME SURPRISES. You can never go wrong adding an element of surprise to an evening. Whether you've just met someone at a bar or are planning your first date, think of ways to show her that you're, well, a little different—and that you like her enough to invest a little energy. *"I met this cute guy who bought me a few drinks, then suggested we take a walk in the park next door,"* a 33-year-old landscaper told us. *"He didn't try to kiss me; we just walked and talked. We got to know each other better than we ever would have just sitting in the bar."*

LIKE HER BEFORE YOU LOVE HER. This one is so obvious that it shouldn't need mentioning, but apparently there are a lot of men out there who equate conquest with seduction and rate their success in the world by the number of women they bed. It's not our place to judge what you do. If you want to act like a horn-dog at full moon, go for it. Just don't be surprised when you get a lot of thoroughly disgusted looks.

Women want men who like them. It's as simple as that. When you're on a first date or approaching a woman to get that first date, concentrate on *her.* Not her cleavage. Not what you're hoping to do later that night. Just her. What she has to say. What she does for a living. What she likes to do on Sunday mornings. The music she likes. If she has kids. Who her friends are. In other words, treat her like a person, not the trophy at the end of the race.

A man who genuinely likes the woman he's with, who shows his appreciation in a hundred different ways, and who doesn't attempt to pressure her into bed is going to get a lot further than the guy whose only intention is to score.

▼

Knights in the Middle Ages practiced having sex by thrusting into goose down, with 30 pounds of stones attached to their hips. The idea of this exercise was to get them into shape so that they could have sex without taking off their heavy armor.

▲

EXPECT NOTHING. If you doubt that women have instincts that are as finely tuned as any signal from the Hubble space telescope, just see how long you last when you start out with pure sexual vibes. She'll know what you're after, probably sooner than you do. She might let you buy her a drink. She might even enjoy flirting for awhile. But you can bet she won't stick around very long.

There's nothing wrong with showing sexual interest. Women like the flirting game every bit as much as men—but only when there's something else behind it. Suppose you're sitting at a bar and decide to send a drink to a woman a few stools down. Do it because it makes you feel good to be generous. Do it because you like the way she looks and want her to notice you. Don't do it because you hope for some kind of instant payoff. Do you really expect torrid sex for the price of a measly margarita? You want the gesture to say, "Yes, I'm interested, but I'm not waiting to pounce."

FOLLOW UP. When you meet a woman for the first time, there will come the hour when you're ready for the next step. It could be backing away if you aren't (or she isn't) interested, or it could be setting up the next date. Once again, confidence goes a long way. Come right out and ask for her phone number or e-mail address.

THE MYTH OF THE SWINGING SINGLE

Married men awash in nostalgia for their sex-filled single days should remind themselves of two things: (1) Memory is an unreliable beast, and (2) their fantasies probably don't jibe very well with reality.

It's true that single men generally have the time and opportunity to meet potential partners, but note the word *potential.* Surveys show that those boring, predictable, stay-at-home married men have a lot more sex than their single counterparts.

The landmark *Sex in America* survey revealed that married men have sex anywhere from three times a week to several times a month. Fewer than half of the single men surveyed reported the same sexual frequency.

"Don't make me nervous by just hanging around and making me wonder if you like me or not," a 27-year-old makeup artist told us. *"Be direct. Say something like, 'I'd like to spend some time with you; is there a time we can get together?'"*

COURTESY COUNTS. Don't ask for her number if you have no intention of calling. You wouldn't like it if someone left you hanging, so don't do it to her. If you are interested, be ready to end the evening on a friendly note. Sure, the attraction might be so strong that you're both eager to tumble into bed, but don't count on it—or give the impression that that's what you're waiting for. You want her to feel liked, not used—and a little anticipation isn't a bad thing.

THE FUN OF FLIRTING

Flirting hovers up among life's top pleasures. And unlike many of today's youthful fashions, it improves over the years. The more you practice it, the more you'll enjoy it. And meeting an accomplished flirt along life's winding road can keep your libido from sinking into the couch and giving up.

Flirting, like the tango, requires two willing partners. Sure, you can flirt endlessly in the face of indifference, but one-sided flirting works about as well as waterskiing behind a bicycle. Find someone who enjoys the game and get on the same page about where you're going with it. Some women (and men) flirt only when they're actively seeking something more. Others flirt simply because they enjoy the subtly charged sexual interaction, with no intention of taking it further. In either case, flirting for the wrong reasons (or mismatched reasons) will leave you both with a faint residue of disappointment.

Flirting can progress by degrees from casual to overtly sexual. There are no rules because everyone enjoys different things. One woman might enjoy flirting that's frankly sexual. For another, it's all about mental interplay charged with that little unspoken something. However, the women we talked to agreed on a few key points.

LESS IS ALWAYS MORE. Guys who flirt overtly the second they meet a woman come across as desperate, not cool. Go ahead and show some interest by making a few playful remarks. Then hold back and see how the woman responds. If she caps your lines with some of her own or quickly moves into more personal territory, consider it a green light to go ahead. Otherwise, back off and give her some space.

DO SOME E-FLIRTING. E-mail is a great flirting tool. Unlike a phone call, it allows a woman to play without feeling hemmed in— or committing to a potentially lousy first date. It gives her a chance to see how your mind works and how you play. At the same time, writing is a more contemplative process than talking. You can easily shift the tone from just-fun flirting to more serious discussions, depending on your mood and what's happening in your life. She'll get a better sense of who you are day to day, not just when you're leaning on a pool table with a drink in your hand.

GO SLOW WITH PHYSICAL FLIRTING. A light touch on the arm, leaning in close when you talk, or picking up her hand to look at her ring are all great forms of flirting that say loud and clear, "I'm interested!" But don't move too fast on the physical gestures. In fact, wait for her to make the first move. Women get hit on all the time. Moving too fast at an early juncture gives the impression that you're more interested in getting into bed than in learning anything about the woman you're with.

LEARN THE SIGNS. Flirting is frequently verbal, but it doesn't have to be. It doesn't even have to be conscious. A lot of erotic interplay occurs just below the level of awareness. Whether you mean to or not, you're constantly beaming signals, and women do the same. Scientists who study body language say that the signals we send don't have the same unequivocal meanings as, say, a sentence in the Sunday paper. But they can still be read with a high degree of certainty. The man who can accurately interpret a woman's body language will have a much better sense of where a relationship is going—or if it is actually going anywhere. Most of these flirtation signals are among 52 common nonverbal behaviors documented in the mid-1980s by researcher Monica M. Moore, Ph.D., of Webster University in St. Louis, who observed more than 200 adults in settings such as bars, restaurants, and parties.

▶ She touches her chin or cheek. She's thinking about the two of you relating in some fashion—though not necessarily sexually. It's a good sign because it means she's taking you seriously.

▶ Her palms are facing you. She's happy to be the one carrying the conversation. Sit back and listen.

CONCEIVE THIS

Unless you've had a vasectomy or your partner is unable to conceive for whatever reason, reliable birth control is always an irksome presence on the sexual scene. Couples resort to all sorts of techniques—and embrace more than a few fallacies—in order to circumvent nature's relentless mandate to procreate.

More than a few couples believe that a woman won't get pregnant if she has her period, if the man uses a condom, or if he withdraws prior to ejaculating. It's true that having sex in each of these circumstances lowers the odds of pregnancy, but it's far from guaranteed.

Sex during menstruation. Sperm can survive for 3 to 5 days when they nestle in the welcoming warmth of the womb. And women with irregular periods or menstrual cycles that are shorter than the average 28 days can ovulate close to the time of menstruation, allowing your sperm to hit pay dirt just when you'd least expect. Also, women with erratic menstrual cycles frequently "spot," or lose small amounts of blood, which can easily be mistaken for a full-blown period. Having unprotected sex during this time can easily leave you with a little bundle of surprise 9 months later.

Using a condom. Used properly, condoms are a very effective form of birth control. Assuming, that is, that they don't slip off or blow up. It happens more often than you might think. There are about 14 pregnancies among every 100 couples who rely on condoms for a year. Put another way, a couple using condoms for 10 years can statistically be expected to have an unintended pregnancy.

Withdrawing before ejaculation. A small amount of seminal fluid, sometimes called pre-come, leaks from the penis before ejaculation—and it contains the same sperm concentration as a full-fledged ejaculation. The failure rate of the so-called withdrawal method is about 20 percent.

▶ She rests an elbow in her palm, with the other palm facing up, or she stretches. She's attentive, but she wants something more from you. This is the time to take charge of the conversation. Don't wait for her; she's done putting out energy for the moment.

▶ She glances at her watch when you pass her—on the street, at a party, wherever. This one's a no-brainer. Time to move on.

▶ Her pupils dilate when she's looking in your eyes, or she raises both eyebrows or blinks rapidly. Keep talking—you have her attention.

▶ She places a fingernail between her teeth or wets her lips with her tongue. Sure, her lips could just be a little dry. But women unconsciously do these things when they're with a man they're interested in.

▶ She plays with keys or jewelry or handles her glass. These signals are a bit ambiguous. We tend to get busy with our hands when we're not entirely focused on the person we're with. On the other hand, it can also mean we're interested but are a bit uncomfortable about interacting too directly. If the woman does these things and also plays with her hair or adjusts her clothing more than once or twice, she's definitely interested.

▶ She sits with her legs slightly apart or crossed; her foot is pointed at you. Very good signs. She's drawing your attention to her legs. She wants you to notice her.

SLOW AND ATTENTIVE:
THE ART OF FOREPLAY

Like stretching before a race, foreplay prepares your body, and your partner's, for the "workout" to come. At its best, it communicates the desire and passion that you feel. You might think that a rapid-fire transition from "Let's go to my house" to "Lights on or off?" adequately expresses your heartfelt romance. Your prospective partner will see it differently.

Foreplay rarely gets the attention it deserves. The word itself suggests that it's merely a prelude to something else, but it can and should be its own erotic reward. It's an essential part of love-making because it equalizes your and your partner's levels of arousal. Most women are slower to kindle than men. All of the courtship, kissing, and touching elevates your partner's arousal to equal yours. When you finally do have intercourse, you'll have the satisfaction of knowing that you're both entering the race from the same place.

A 23-year-old law student in Wilmington, Delaware, put it best. *"Foreplay! I want to really, really want sex. He needs to kiss me and caress me in sensual places, especially my back or neck. I'm also a sucker for repeatedly being told that he thinks I'm gorgeous. That encourages me to be more open and free about my sexuality."*

The best foreplay goes beyond two bodies in a bed. It starts long before you take off your clothes and lasts, well, as long as you care to keep it burning. Every woman, like every man, has very different sexual desires. But nearly all of the women we talked to look for a few similar things.

KEEP IT HOT. Men tend to jump straight from erotic thoughts into sexual action. For women, anticipation plays a much greater role. The brain, remember, is the ultimate erogenous zone. If you wait until after Jay Leno's monologue to start some foreplay, the ensuing sex, assuming there is any, will be perfunctory at best. You'll enjoy yourself a lot more if you kick it into gear long before it's time for sex. Send her a quick e-mail at work saying you're thinking about her. Leave a sexy voice mail. Rub her feet while you're watching the news. The more relaxed and desired you make her feel, the higher her sexual energy will climb.

ENGAGE THE SENSES. Light a scented candle. Pour her a glass of wine. Rub her legs. Put a rose on her pillow. Whisper those sweet nothings that we all like to hear. You'll notice, by the way, that we haven't said a thing about watching her get undressed or popping in a sexy DVD. Ramped-up eroticism can certainly be a part of fore-play, but it's hardly the only part. Save them until later. Relaxing with preliminaries as though you have all the time in the world—and whether or not you're actually planning to have sex—creates a romantic ambience that's the ultimate aphrodisiac.

FIND HER ZONES. *All* of them. Too many men approach fore-play as some perfunctory kisses, a quick rub of the breasts, and some exploratory attention to the genitals prior to the eager leap aboard. The best foreplay is a whole-body experience, and her erogenous zones, like yours, deserve to be explored.

FORGET THE UNAPPETIZING NAME. Erogenous zones are simply clusters of nerve endings that lie just below the surface of the skin. The genital area is loaded with them, but they're found throughout the body—and these bean-size areas are exquisitely sen-sitive to touch. Stimulating the nerves sends electrical signals blasting into the brain's pleasure centers.

A previous lover may have loved to have her neck kissed and sucked. Your current partner may or may not respond the same way. Don't depend on prior experience to guide your hands. If you pay attention, you'll soon discover the exact areas that make your lover tingle—and she'll undoubtedly do the same for you. Think of it as a search for the New World, with plenty of surprises along the way. These are the most common erogenous zones.

▶ Breasts. They're pretty much a universal hot spot for men as well as women. Don't go straight for the nipple (unless she asks you to). For most women, the spots slightly above both breasts and the area in the middle are wonderfully sensitive.

The nipple is certainly a pleasure zone, but it's often *too* sensitive in the early stages of lovemaking.

▶ **Mouth.** Kiss her as much as you like to be kissed. Explore with your tongue. Put your fingers in her mouth and let her suck them.

▶ **Abdomen.** Kiss and touch the areas 2 to 3 inches on either side of her navel.

▶ **Fingers and toes.** Rub them, pull on them, put them in your mouth.

▶ **Arms, wrists, and underarms.** Stroke very lightly with your fingertips. Extend her arm slightly and stroke all the way up into the hollow of her armpit. Vary your touch by using your fingertips, stroking feather-light or a little stronger. Smother her arm with kisses.

▶ **Back.** Rub out the tension in her shoulders with some firm squeezes. Press your thumbs down either side of her spine. Pay particular attention to her lower back. It's loaded with nerve endings.

▶ **Buttocks.** Use the heels of your hands and press firmly. Concentrate on the spots on the outer curve of her flanks. You'll probably find an arousal spot about two-thirds of the way down each of the cheeks, slightly toward the outer edge. Throw in a few playful nips or spanks if she likes a little more force.

▶ **Ears.** Concentrate on the lobes and outer curves. Don't just jam your tongue into her ear, although many women like that as well. Whisper very softly into her ear. Even if she can't hear what you're saying, the softness of your breath will feel very pleasant.

▶ Feet. Rub them thoroughly with oil. It's deeply relaxing and very, very sensual. Massage or suck her toes and deeply rub the soles. Both areas are loaded with hot spots.

▶ Head. Gently stroking her eyebrows, around her eye sockets, and the hollows beneath her cheekbones will stimulate the release of feel-good endorphins.

▶ Knees. The backs of the knees, like the soles of the feet, contain an enormous number of nerve endings.

▶ Legs. Stroke the entire length, starting at her ankles and moving all the way up. Pause at her knees, then pay extra attention to her inner thighs with touches and kisses. Take your time. Her anticipation will keep climbing as you move higher—holding back, moving higher, teasing and touching.

▶ Back of the neck. The feel of your breath or tongue on this very sensitive area will send shivers down her spine. Press the spot where the back of her neck meets her skull to release tension and stress.

▶ Stomach. Use a circular motion to rub her belly. Run your hands from her waist down the inside curve of her hips toward her genitals.

▶ Wrists. The smooth skin below the palm is very sensitive. She'll enjoy just about any gentle sensation here—fingertips, lips, breath.

A final word on pleasure spots. Men tend to prefer a rougher touch than women. Don't touch her the way you'd want her to touch you. Each spot responds differently to stimulation. Try different pressures and touches, using your fingers, lips, tongue, and breath. Sensitivity will also vary depending on your partner's level of arousal. Nibbling her earlobe might fire her up during foreplay but elicit little response once you've entered her. Play, and keep playing. You'll discover soon enough exactly what she likes.

SENSUAL MASSAGE

Back when we ran around in skins and ate gritty roots and raw meat, our vocabulary wasn't very impressive. Men, trying their best, probably courted their partners by looking deeply into their eyes and saying things like "urghgh" and "mmphh." These tender expressions of love didn't get them very far, so they depended on their hands to touch and caress. That worked a little better, as evidenced by the fact that we're here today.

In today's world, though, words permeate every facet of our lives. We've almost forgotten how to use our hands and bodies to give the most potent messages of all, the ones that say "I care about you," and "Let's share this moment."

Some experts suggest that massage is second only to herbal medicine as the oldest form of physical therapy. Every time scientists study the effects of massage, they come away impressed. It improves mood and reduces stress, anxiety, and tension. That's no small thing when you're trying to incorporate more sensual pleasure into your life. Researchers at the Touch Research Institute at the University of Miami found that massage causes a decline in three different stress hormones. They also found that couples who share massages experience less anxiety about sexual performance and have more physical intimacy.

Massage stimulates the senses, and that makes it a natural adjunct to good sex. Sensual massage soothes at the same time that it arouses and communicates warmth and love. It can also tell you a lot about your partner's physical, mental, and emotional moods. Those neck and shoulder muscles that get all bunched up from sitting at a desk; the sighs of pleasure as tension melts away under your fingers; the spontaneous arousal from skin-on-skin connections.

Massage isn't only about hands, of course. You can rub each other with your arms, thighs, stomach, and buttocks—with any part of your body, in fact. How do you transform a stress-easing massage into one that communicates pure sexual energy? Here are a few things you may want to try.

TOUCH AND TALK. The best massages take place in silence, except for the occasional happy sigh or moan. But when you and your partner first start rubbing each other right, keep the talk going. Don't try to guess what feels good. Ask her. Have her tell you what touches she likes best. Whether she wants you to start at this part of the body or over there. Whether long and soft trumps deep and hard.

HIT THE SWITCH. Sure, you can have a great massage under 100-watt incandescents. Why not get a checkup while you're at it? Massage is all about relaxation and erotic play. So flip the dimmer switch or light a few candles. You and your partner will be less self-conscious and much more relaxed when you're framed by sexy twilight.

OIL UP YOUR MOOD. Get oils made specifically for massage. They tend to be lighter than other oils. You can still feel skin on skin, but your fingers will glide more sensuously, without rough friction.

There are literally dozens of massage oils to choose from. Most people like an oil with just a hint of scent—not only because it smells good but also because different scents stimulate the body and mind in different ways. These are some of the most popular.

▶ Anise has a stimulating licorice scent reputed to enhance sexual desire.

▶ Cardamom's sharp, sweet scent is believed to be an aphrodisiac for men as well as women.

▶ Cinnamon is the ultimate comfort spice—and studies show that it has a pronounced effect on a man's libido.

▶ Clove's pungent spiciness energizes and enhances any erotic experience.

▶ Jasmine, also called Queen of the Night, promotes feelings of love and sensuality. It's a great choice for those warm, full-moon nights.

▶ Myrrh contains chemical compounds that have molecular structures similar to testosterone's.

▶ Orange blossom is a traditional favorite at weddings, for obvious reasons: The heady yet refreshing scent is a natural for lovemaking.

▶ Patchouli's musky allure is traditionally thought to represent the scent of sex itself.

▶ Rose is probably the most popular scent in the world. It inspires feelings of love and sexuality.

Once you've selected your oil, it's time to put your hands to work. (Rub the oil between your palms for a few seconds to warm it up.) Bookstores almost always stock several books on sensual massage techniques, but it isn't rocket science. You'll learn more by practicing on your partner and listening to her sighs than you'll glean from a dozen expensive books.

The most important thing is to keep your hands in contact with her body all the time. Don't dispel the mood by lifting your hands to answer the phone. This isn't the time to take a sip from a glass of ice water unless you warm your hands afterward. Technique isn't as important as taking your time. Still, there are a few classic massage moves that are perfect for the sensual touch.

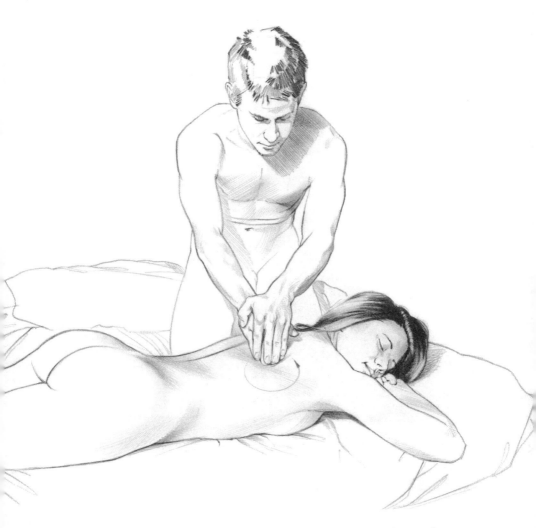

▶ Circling. Put one hand on top of the other and make small, firm circles up and down her body.

▶ Swimming. Use both hands to make separate circles, moving them in opposite directions. Bring them close together, then stroke up and away, as though doing the breaststroke. This technique is especially good when massaging the back, thighs, and buttocks.

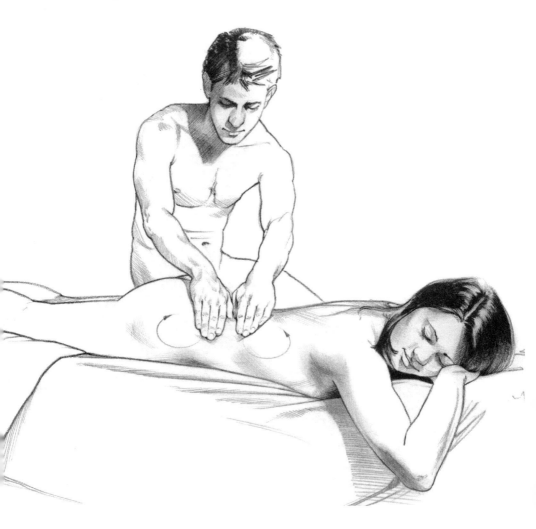

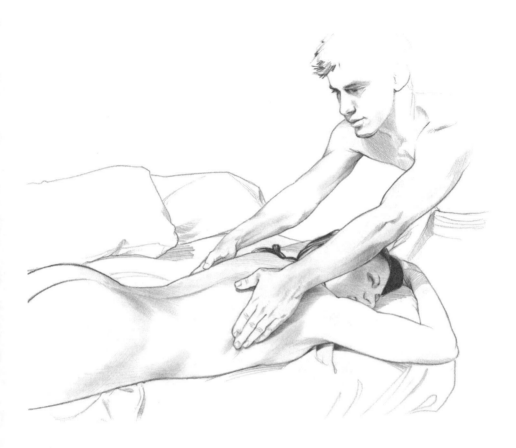

▶ Effleurage. This is a very sensual stroke that follows the contours of your partner's body. Press gently, outlining muscles as you go. Trace the muscles in her back and the curves of her breasts and stomach. Or sit on her thighs as she lies on her stomach. Put your palms on her buttocks, fingers pointing toward her head, and press firmly and smoothly in slow circles.

▶ Thumb love. Use both your thumbs, alternating pressure from one to the other as you press on either side of her spine.

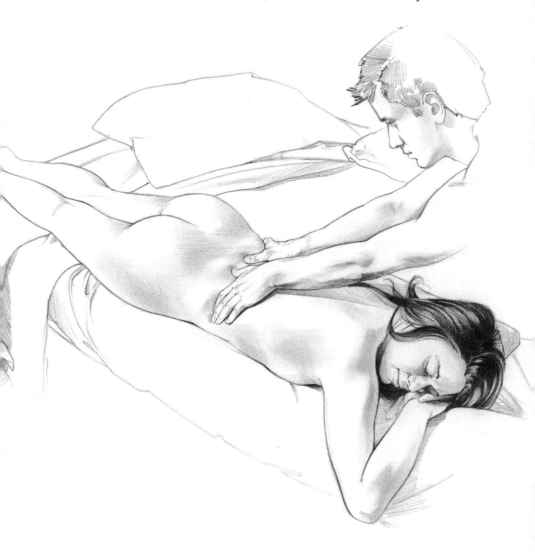

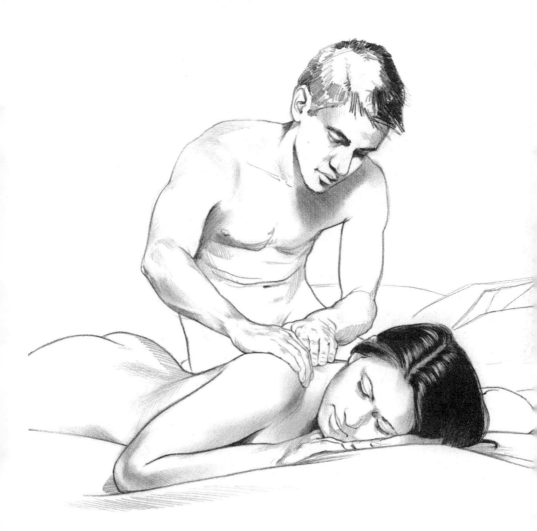

▶ Feathering. Run your hands as lightly as possible over your partner's body—so lightly that they feel more like a whisper than a touch.

THE TEASE THAT PLEASES

It's too bad that teasing has such a bad reputation. It can be a great deal of fun when you're priming the sexual pump. Obviously, we're not talking about schoolyard teasing, where the object is to verbally pummel and then shun the poor kids who never made it into the "in" group—which is to say, just about all of us. Sexual teasing is a whole different ball game.

Think about the little shivers of excitement that you get when a flirtatious somebody at a party or a bar sidles up to you, runs her hand down your back, then mysteriously disappears to who knows where. Now imagine the same scenario with one key difference: She actually sticks around after you start to burn—and continues the adventure with all sorts of fun and games.

Teasing basically means getting each other as hot and bothered as you possibly can, but not all at once—slowly, with patience and self-control. The goal is to arouse each other to a pure state of heat, then deny and delay the inevitable until you're almost begging for

CIRCUMCISION: GOOD OR BAD FOR SEX?

Most male newborns in the United States are circumcised. But in the past few years, the ancient procedure has gotten increasingly bad press—not only because of the pain it causes the infant but also because some advocates believe that removing the foreskin dulls sexual sensation.

New research suggests it isn't so. Scientists at the Louisiana School of Medicine studied 15 men who were circumcised as adults and found that they experienced no less satisfaction than they did before. Nor were there any significant changes in their sex drive or ability to have an erection.

The American Academy of Pediatrics no longer recommends routine circumcision for boys because it doesn't confer any medical benefits. But if you've already been circumcised, so be it. It won't affect your love life.

sex. You're taking the scenic route rather than the freeway. Starting to kiss, then pulling away. Touching here, but not quite *there*. If you do it right, you'll keep withholding, denying, tantalizing, and circling closer until she truly *must* be touched. Delayed gratification can bring out the best in both of you; restraint, in other words, pays great dividends.

You need three things to be a great tease: imagination, attention to her responses, and a totally unhurried buildup to the finale. The element of surprise will also work in your favor, especially if you've been together for awhile. She knows your routines as well as you know hers. So offer up a new menu now and then.

DO YOUR ADVANCE WORK. Tell her ahead of time how you plan to seduce her. Don't tell her everything, just enough to get her thinking. For example, that you're going to meet her at the door, pull her close, and run your tongue around her neck. How you'll be thinking truly nasty thoughts all day. How the very thought of touching her breasts makes you totally aroused.

DON'T GET CARRIED AWAY AND SPILL EVERYTHING. The idea is to tease her, not to spend the day regaling her with explicit dirty talk. Say less; imply more. Don't worry; her imagination will meet you halfway.

TOUCH HER HOW (AND WHERE) SHE LEAST EXPECTS IT. If you usually stroke her breasts with your fingers, taste them with your tongue instead. Caress her thighs in an unexpected direction. Stop, then start again—or not. Keep her guessing.

WORK FROM BEHIND. "Blind" teasing is a fantastic turn-on. Stand behind her so she can't see you and won't know what to expect. If you really want to throw her expectations out the window, cover her eyes with a silk handkerchief. Stand behind her, beside her, in front of her, moving and touching in unexpected ways. Don't scare her with sudden movements, though. Keep your touches gentle and slow.

GIVE HER WHAT SHE WANTS—BUT JUST FOR AWHILE. As she gets more and more worked up, for example, spend some time caressing one of her favorite spots. Keep doing it until her erotic energy is almost over the top. Then stop, totally stop. Kiss her on the lips and ask if she'd like you to touch her anywhere in particular. When she tells you, go ahead and touch the area oh-so-lightly, maybe even with just your breath. Move to another spot, then come back to the "good" spot again and give it a little more.

PLAY THIS GAME FOR HOURS. When you're both so hot that you can hardly stand it, enter her with just the tip of your penis, moving it gently and withholding the full thrust. If she tries to pull you deeper inside, resist and pull back. Keep playing, going a little farther each time. When you finally do find yourselves making full-fledged love, you'll both be way beyond ready—and this night might turn out to be the one that you talk about ("Do you remember when . . .") for months to come.

CHAPTER 3

BETTER SEX TECHNIQUE:
A REFRESHER COURSE

**NO SELF-RESPECTING GUY NEEDS LESSONS IN BED-
ROOM BASICS, AND YOU'RE NO EXCEPTION. EXCEPT,
WELL, WHAT DOES YOUR PARTNER THINK?** It can't hurt to
review what she wants you to know about her body and her orgasm. And positions? You think you've tried them all? You'll be surprised by the variations we came up with.

KNOW THE TERRITORY

We begin our lives as women. Every fetus is female until about 8
weeks or so. It's only after the male genes send out the signal for
testosterone that the embryonic labia develop into a scrotum, and
the clitoris transforms into a penis. Thus you emerge, some months
later, a boy.

Your brief life as a woman hardly gave you enough time to really
get acquainted with those private parts that are so different from

yours. Unless you're truly bold in the bedroom and have a very pa-tient partner along with a four-cell Maglite, you've probably never explored a woman's genitals with clinical precision. That's okay. As one woman told us, *"You don't need a road map to find ground zero."*

Still, uncertainty about the terrain is not at all uncommon. A woman's body can indeed seem mysterious, to her as well as to you. In lovemaking, the more you know about a woman's intricacies—which, compared with a man's external inches of anatomy, are more or less hidden—the more pleasure you'll be able to give as well as receive.

Your partners don't expect you to be a gynecologist. You can be a perfectly good lover without knowing the scientific names for a woman's bits and pieces. But you'll still want to get a handle on the lay of the land, as it were. Moving from the outside in, here's what you'll find.

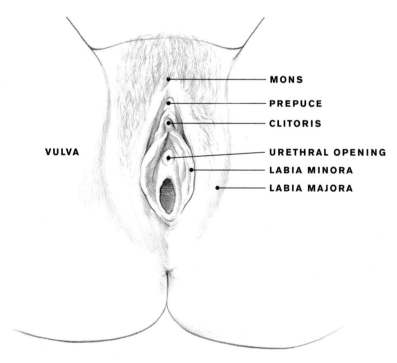

MONS
PREPUCE
CLITORIS
VULVA
URETHRAL OPENING
LABIA MINORA
LABIA MAJORA

The exterior portion, known collectively as the *vulva,* includes the soft mound *(mons)* over the pelvic bone.

The outer lips, *labia majora,* extend from the mons to below the opening of the vagina. The lips consist of a fold of skin on each side, which is filled with fatty tissue, nerve endings, and sweat and oil glands. These lips generally cover the vaginal opening, although they open up somewhat when a woman is aroused.

The inner lips, *labia minora,* lie inside the outer lips. They extend from just above the clitoris to below the vaginal opening. The inner lips are thinner and possess more nerve endings than the outer lips. The term *inner* is somewhat misleading because they commonly protrude beyond the outer lips.

Both the inner and outer lips come in many different shapes, sizes, and colors, just as men's penises do. These portions of a woman's genitals may be red, pink, purple, or black and may even change color during arousal.

The clitoral hood, or *prepuce,* lies just below the place where the inner lips meet at the peak. The hood is a small piece of skin that's the female version of the foreskin.

Today, we make oaths by putting our hands on our hearts. In biblical days, men did it by putting their hands on their penises.

The clitoris, the most sensitive part of the genitals, is a woman's key to orgasm. Some have described the clitoris as button shaped—but that would be a mighty small button. "Tiny dot" is more like it. "Where the hell *is* the damn thing?" is a question asked by more than a few frustrated men.

In truth, the clitoris is small, but not that small. Just as much of your penis is buried inside your body, much of the clitoris is similarly concealed. The body of the clitoris, which is as big as the joint of your thumb, lies entirely out of sight underneath the clitoral tip, the part that you can touch.

Branching off the clitoral body are two clitoral branches, or legs, that flare backward into the body, running near the ends of the muscles that line the inner thighs. This is part of the reason that stroking a woman's thighs feels so good to her. The legs also stretch underneath the labia, so stimulating that area indirectly stimulates the clitoris.

When a woman is aroused, her pelvic region fills with blood, and the clitoris pulls back against the pubic bone. At the same time, the labia swell, which makes the clitoris appear erect. Paradoxically, the clitoris can all but disappear underneath the prepuce when a woman is highly stimulated.

SEX FOR THE HEART

It makes for great barroom conversation when some high-society luminary is reported to have died in the sack, usually in the company of a woman 30 years younger. More than a few men have left the Earth in this memorable fashion, but your chances of dying at any given time are actually lower if you enjoy a lively sex life.

It's true that men who have sex frequently are somewhat more likely to suffer a heart attack or stroke in the midst of sex than those who indulge less often, according to a report in the *Journal of Epidemiology and Community Health.* However, research suggests that men who are active in bed are less likely overall to die from cardiovascular causes.

Researchers report that men who have sex three or four times a week may be able to cut their risk of stroke or a major heart attack in half. One study found that men who had two or more orgasms a week were about half as likely to die prematurely as those who had one orgasm a month.

It may be that sexually active men are healthier to begin with, but scientists also speculate that men who have frequent sex are giving themselves healthful cardiovascular workouts at the same time.

The urinary opening, the *urethra,* lies just below the clitoral tip.

The vagina, the place where you put your penis, is a sort of barrel 3 to 4 inches long. (To completely fill the vagina, a man needs to be only about an inch longer than the vaginal canal. That's why all of the male wishful thinking about having a larger penis is pretty much beside the point.) You can't really see it because it's all internal.

The vagina is mainly muscle, covered with ribs (that you can feel) and a mucus-producing surface similar to the lining of the mouth. The vaginal walls normally close in on each other. When a woman is excited, though, the walls expand, and slippery lubricant is produced. She gets wet, in other words. This doesn't necessarily mean she wants to have sex right away, just that her body is preparing for it.

The fabled G-spot is named after Ernst Grafenberg, M.D., who discovered this rough, dime-size patch of skin in the 1950s. It's gen-

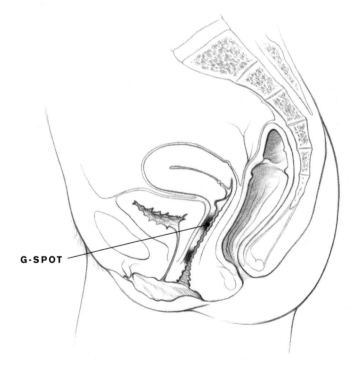

G-SPOT

erally located on the vaginal wall about 2 to 3 inches past and behind the pubic bone—but it's not found in the same place in all women. Stimulating the G-spot can, in some women, produce intense arousal or orgasm. Others find that the G-spot is no more sensitive than any other part of the vagina. In fact, doctors estimate that fewer than 10 percent of women even know where it is. It's hardly the Holy Grail of sexual satisfaction. It's worth asking your partner to help you find it, or if it even matters. In some women, stimulating this spot causes ejaculation—an outpouring from the paraurethral glands located on either side of the urethra.

There are a few more hot spots you'll want to know about. The anterior fornix zone lies deep within the vagina, above the G-spot and near the cervix (the neck of the uterus). Some women experience great pleasure when they're stroked in the area between the G-spot and the anterior fornix. While you're at it, take a moment to explore the perineum, the patch of smooth, usually hairless skin between the vagina and anus. It's exquisitely sensitive, in men as well as women.

THE FEMALE ORGASM

A woman's sexual responses are far more complicated than a man's—so much so, in fact, that doctors aren't sure exactly what a female orgasm is. Sex researchers William Masters, M.D., and Virginia Johnson, in their methodical way, described orgasm as the third phase of a woman's sexual response cycle.

▶ 1. Excitement: The genitals start filling with blood and she starts producing vaginal lubrication.

▶ 2. Plateau: Muscular tension increases and the tissues continue filling with blood. Breathing rate increases, the skin flushes, and the vagina swells.

THE QUEST FOR
SIMULTANEOUS ORGASM

For some mysterious reason, the simultaneous orgasm has become a symbol of both a couple's level of intimacy and a man's sexual competence. Sex therapists say that it's not unusual for couples with great sex lives to feel that they're somehow missing out because they rarely or never come at the same time.

Welcome to the real world. It's rare for any two people, however long they've been together and whatever their level of sexual expertise, to get aroused at precisely the same time. It's certainly possible to come together, especially when you're familiar with each other's timing and rhythms. But count on it? Not a good idea.

Nor should it. Timing orgasms, like counting them, is a task best left to researchers, not lovers. Besides, coming together means that you're too out of your head to closely watch your lover get lost in orgasm. Who wants to miss that?

▶ 3. Orgasm: Muscular tension is suddenly released, and blood starts to exit the genitals. The uterus and vagina contract at 0.08-second intervals—the same rate of contraction experienced by men during their orgasms. Some women have post-orgasm contractions that can persist to some degree for up to 24 hours.

▶ 4. Resolution: The body returns to its prearoused state.

One of the primary reasons that women are more likely than men to have multiple orgasms is that the blood tends to remain in the pelvic area much longer. After a woman comes, her body is more likely to retreat to the second, plateau stage rather than fall all the way back to stage one, the way men do. It's easier to achieve a second orgasmic peak when you aren't starting from scratch.

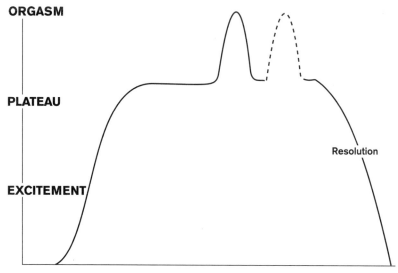

Female Sexual Response Cycle
(shown with possible second orgasm)

Not all women are multi-orgasmic, incidentally. Many come once; then they're done. However, sex researcher Alfred Kinsey, Ph.D., reported that the vast majority of women he studied did have the capacity for multiple orgasms. That doesn't mean that all of them do it, however, or even want to. Some women are too sensitive after they come to resume sexual activity. Others are happy to stop when their men do.

It's one of nature's paradoxes that nearly all men can have orgasms from intercourse alone, but only about 30 percent of women respond the same way. Most women need direct clitoral stimulation, which happens only marginally during intercourse. Couples who spend enough time together invariably explore a host of pleasurable ways to supplement their lovemaking with direct clitoral contact. A man might touch his partner during or after intercourse. Or she'll do it herself. Don't let shyness get in the way—and definitely don't assume that you somehow failed if she touches herself. It's part of the reality of female sexuality. Besides, most men enjoy watching women get themselves off—and can pick up a few tips along the way.

"I need a lot of reassurance from him that he thinks I'm beautiful and sexy," a 28-year-old Chicago insurance broker told us. *"That will give me the confidence to be more brazen in bed—and to feel comfortable masturbating while he watches."*

HANDS-ON PLEASURE

A theme that you've undoubtedly noticed running through this book is that there's never a *best* way when it comes to sex. Women are wildly different in what they like, just as men are. You can make a career of reading sex books and watching sexy movies, and at the end of the day, all you really know is what *some* women like, not necessarily what *your* woman likes.

Still, there are some general approaches to a woman's body that tend to give the most pleasure, most of the time. One thing you can be sure of is that her physical responses won't be the same as yours. It's the difference that makes life exciting!

TOUCH HER GENTLY. Generalizations rarely work, but this is a good fallback position. Women are far more likely than men to respond to light touches, certainly at first, when things are heating up. Pay attention to her body language: If she pushes herself hard against your hand, for example, you'll know a little more pressure will be welcome. Don't depend on body language alone, however. Ask her what she likes. Ask her to move your hand just the way she wants it. "Do you like it when I do this?" "What would feel best right now?" "A little more pressure?" Too many couples make love in total silence, which can result in endless sexual guessing games.

LICK YOUR FINGERS. Or moisten them with your partner's secretions. Use a lubricant. The vaginal tissues are much more sensitive than the tough skin on the penis. Women need moisture and lubrication to be comfortable.

START IN THE "BONE" POSITION. Lie beside your partner and rest the heel of your hand and wrist on the mons, the bony area

DO MEN REALLY
RUN FROM COMMITMENT?

It's certainly true that some men will commit to nothing more serious than getting a woman into bed. It's also true that young men who are in only their second or third "serious" relationships probably don't want to start discussing toasters. But there's nothing in a man's genetic makeup that makes him inherently unstable in the relationship department.

Look at it this way. A man who spends substantial amounts of time with a woman has already, in his mind, made quite a commitment. If nothing else, he's choosing to hang around with her rather than spend time in so-called male activities, such as throwing popcorn at the TV or getting blind drunk with his buddies at the corner bar.

When you get right down to it, most men want the same things as women: friendship, someone to count on, and, of course, regular sex.

where the pubic hair begins. Your partner will almost certainly want more than cursory attention, and anchoring your wrist will help prevent your arm from tiring too easily.

START WITH CIRCLES. Move your finger or fingers in gentle circles on top of the genitals—the lips as well as the clitoris; it's a movement most women really like. Back and forth is fine, too, especially if you alternate it with circular moves.

COVER A BROAD AREA, THEN FOCUS IN. Don't spend too much time on the clitoris at first. It can be too sensitive if you hit it right away. Start with broad strokes, slowly narrowing the area of stimulation as her pleasure builds. Use your index and middle fingers to lightly surround the clitoral ridge and tip. Move your fingers in circles or up and down—the motions a woman often uses to stimulate herself.

TOUCH INDIRECTLY. Rather than stimulating the clitoris directly, you can curve your fingers around the outer lips and press them gently inward as you massage and stroke. The pressure will gently stimulate the clitoris rather than overstimulating it, and your partner will enjoy the heat radiating from your hand. Slipping a finger into the vagina while you rub the external parts will provide a very pleasurable extra.

PUT YOUR THUMB TO WORK. Insert it inside the vagina and move it in a circular motion. The thumb is stronger than your fingers and won't tire during lengthy sessions. You can also use it to curve into the vagina to stimulate the G-spot.

There are almost infinite variations of each of these moves, many of which you've certainly discovered for yourself. For example, some women love it when a man gently "spins" the clitoris betweens his thumb and forefinger. Or the sensation of having several fingers shimmy in and out of the vagina. Or the feeling of pressure from one hand on the belly while the other hand is in the vagina or on the clitoris.

The bottom line? You'll give your partner the most pleasure when you use the same kinds of motions that she uses herself when masturbating. Don't leave it all to guesswork. Encourage her to tell you, step by step, what feels good, when to keep going, when to try something else. She knows what she wants and will probably welcome encouragement from you to share all.

Which is not to say that all women are verbally forthcoming. As this 27-year-old film technician told us, *"Don't make me talk about it. Just listen and pay attention when I respond to something with little noises or moans or something. I'm not going to say, 'I want you to pull my hair and bite me and bend me over.' If you notice that I seem to get excited when you do a little of that stuff, just keep going."*

ORAL LOVE

Your mouth can create more sensations on your lover's skin than any other part of your body. Most women agree that what makes them most aroused, in fantasy and fact, is oral sex—receiving as well as giving. But the sheer intimacy of oral sex, especially for women, can be intimidating. They've grown up hearing crude jokes about their smell or taste. Even women who love it when a man licks and tastes them often admit that they wonder how much the guys really enjoy it. Trust and comfort play a far greater role than technique. If your partner isn't absolutely secure in her body—and how you respond to her body—oral sex will invariably produce more anxiety than pleasure.

> "I regret to say that we of the FBI are powerless to act in cases of oral/genital intimacy, unless it has in some way obstructed interstate commerce."
>
> —attributed to former FBI director J. EDGAR HOOVER

Let's back up a few steps. The vagina is self-maintaining and self-regulating as well as self-cleaning. Some women do have strong odors, just as some men do. The aroma is distinctive but not at all unpleasant. If you pay attention, you'll notice that the taste of a woman changes often, depending on factors such as diet and alcohol intake. The changes are subtle, though, and in any case, most men find the smell and taste highly arousing. You should certainly feel free to suggest showering before sex. You can probably use one yourself.

There's no great mystery to oral sex. Any touch from your mouth is likely to be pleasurable. You can heighten the pleasure even more with a few basic steps.

COMPLIMENT HER. Women with new partners often feel vulnerable during oral sex and a little bit insecure. One of the most important things you can do, and the sexiest, is praise her throughout. Tell her how good she tastes, how good she makes you feel. Your arousal will heighten hers, and she'll find it much easier to let go when she knows that you're enjoying it as much as she is.

SHALLOW BEATS DEEP. If you're like most of us, your natural instinct is to probe your partner's vagina with your tongue. There's nothing wrong with using your tongue as a sort of surrogate penis, but keep in mind that there are relatively few nerve endings in the vaginal canal itself. Your partner will get a lot more pleasure when you use your whole mouth, not just your tongue, and when you focus your ministrations more on the exterior portions than merely going deep.

TEASE AND DELAY. The clitoris needs plenty of attention, but you don't necessarily want to start there; a woman needs time to get there. You might start by flicking your tongue along her inner thighs, dipping it into her vagina, then passing it across her clitoris. Use your warm, full mouth on the outer parts of her genitals, then back off and concentrate somewhere else. Intermittent sensations tend to be more pleasurable, at least in the early stages, than going full bore on one spot.

SLIDE ALONG THE SIDES. Some women are more sensitive on one side of the clitoris than the other. Try both and check her response—and ask if she has a preference. Sliding your tongue in broad strokes along either side of her clitoris is sometimes more arousing than hitting it full on.

PLAY WITH POSITIONS AND APPROACHES. There are plenty to choose from. Here are a few.

▶ Your head between your partner's legs. This is the classic position, and it makes it easy for you to use your hands as well as your mouth. It also allows the woman to watch what you're doing, which can be a great visual turn-on. The only real drawback is that the woman is pretty much stuck in a passive position because she can't play with your body at the same time. Placing a pillow under your partner's buttocks or under your chest can make it easier for you to move freely.

▶ Encourage your partner to stimulate her clitoris while you lick and suck the lips and run your tongue into the opening.

▶ Slip a finger into her anus while giving oral sex. It's not for everyone, but many women find the extra sensation very exciting. (After contact with the anal area, always wash your hands with soap and water before touching the vulva or vagina.)

▶ The "69" position allows both of you to take an active role. Side by side is the most common configuration; you can also lie on top of her or have her lie on top of you.

▶ Another popular position is to lie on your back while the woman kneels over your face. It puts her in more of an active role, which many women prefer. It's also a comfortable position for men because it puts no strain on the neck, and your hands are free to roam.

▶ A variation of the woman-on-top position is to have her turn around so that her bottom is facing your face.

▶ You can sit up while your partner lays her thighs across your shoulders and locks her ankles behind your head. You hold her tightly by the waist, occasionally letting your hands move across her body.

▶ Your partner can sit in a chair or on the side of the bed while you kneel in front of her. Women often like this position because they can see exactly what the man is doing.

▶ Lie perpendicular to your partner and use back-and-forth movements with your mouth and tongue. Researchers in sex laboratories report that women given oral sex in this position often experience very rapid and intense orgasms.

In their landmark *Sex in America* survey, Chicago researchers found that 83 percent of men ages 18 to 44 enjoyed being on the receiving end of oral sex. (Yeah, you didn't need us to tell you that.)

Unfortunately, their female counterparts aren't always so enthusiastic about the subject. The same survey revealed that 43 percent of women were less than thrilled about performing fellatio. Though you certainly should never push your partner to perform sexual acts that make her uncomfortable, there are steps you can take that may warm her up to what the ancient Chinese called "playing the flute."

As is always the case with anything sexual, the most effective door opener is communication. Your partner may have ingrained inhibitions regarding oral sex. She may have been taught that it's dirty. Or she's afraid of gagging or that you'll ejaculate in her mouth. Her unwillingness may also be simple performance anxiety. By having an open discussion about oral sex, you can get to the heart of her reluctance. Here are some steps for addressing these common concerns.

ADDRESS EJACULATION. There's more to this issue than "spit or swallow." Your partner may not want you to come in her mouth at all. You can assuage her concerns by agreeing to give her a signal, like squeezing her shoulder, when you're about to come. At that point, she's in control, and she can remove your penis from her mouth and use her hand or do whatever makes her most comfortable. Of course, wearing a condom will make this a nonissue.

GO SLOW AND GENTLE. *Deep Throat* may have been a sexy film, but it probably did more harm than good to the perception of oral sex. Your partner may be afraid that she needs to perform like Linda Lovelace and "swallow" your penis to give you pleasure. Or she's afraid you'll start thrusting, and she'll start gagging. Assure her that sucking the head of your penis while stroking the shaft with her hand is a perfectly fine way to perform fellatio and that there's no pressure for her to do anything that makes her uncomfortable.

OFFER TO GO FIRST. The best sex involves giving and re-ceiving. Sometimes all it takes to warm your partner to an idea is for you to offer to do it first. If you perform oral sex on her and she loves it, there's a good chance she will be willing to return the favor. Just remember, this isn't a football game; it's not about keeping score. If she is still reluctant, give her time and continue to enjoy the sexual relationship you have.

SPICE IT UP. You can make fellatio more savory—literally—by adding a flavored oil- or water-based lubricant. A little cool mint or warm cinnamon may increase the appeal of oral sex for her.

ENJOY IT SAFELY. Finally, remember that fellatio is one of the most efficient ways of transmitting the AIDS virus, because blood and semen are the two bodily fluids with the highest concentration of HIV. If don't know your HIV status, wear a condom even during oral sex.

THE SEXY 6 ▶

HABIT IS A POWERFUL THING. MOST OF US SETTLE INTO A COMFORTABLE PATTERN OF SEXUAL POSITIONS AND THEN KEEP DOING THEM, YEAR AFTER YEAR. It makes sense to do what you like, and if you and your partner really prefer, say, the woman-on-top position, there's no compelling reason to change. Unless, of course, you're starting to hanker for something new. In which case, why limit yourself?

You can go a little crazy once you start exploring the different ways men and women can fit together. Some of the sexual positions that you see in erotic manuals or porn flicks look so uncomfortable that it's hard to imagine why anyone bothers. Others require a degree of athleticism that few of us can match. A few take a surprising amount of work to achieve. Hey, sex is supposed to be fun, not work. When you're looking to shake up your sex life, simple beats pretzel every time.

Once you strip away the subtle variations, there are six basic positions for having sex: man on top, woman on top, side by side, sitting, standing, and rear entry. Each has advantages and disadvantages, such as deeper penetration, more body-to-body contact, or ease of performing when you're tired. But why make it complicated? Most couples choose a certain sexual position, or a variety of them, for no other reason than they like them—although physical changes (such as her pregnancy or your back pain) may shift your preferences one way or another.

You're already familiar with the basic positions (illustrated over the next 32 pages), but it might be useful to know what makes each one unique—in terms of comfort, what gets stimulated, how men and women respond, and so on. You'll also discover a few variations that you may want to try.

POSITION #1: MAN ON TOP

It's probably the most popular sexual position in this country because it allows face-to-face intimacy and full-body contact and permits deep thrusts and full penetration. It's comfortable for the woman because she can lie on her back, with or without a pillow to change the angle; men like it because they can control the timing and penetration.

There are a few drawbacks, however. This "missionary position" can be too arousing for men in some cases, causing too-quick ejaculation. A small woman with a bulky partner may find his weight uncomfortable unless he takes care to support his weight on his arms. From a man's point of view, it can be tiring because he's doing most of the heavy lifting.

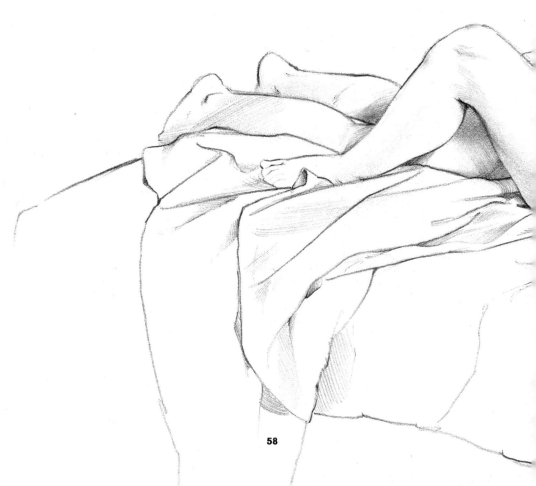

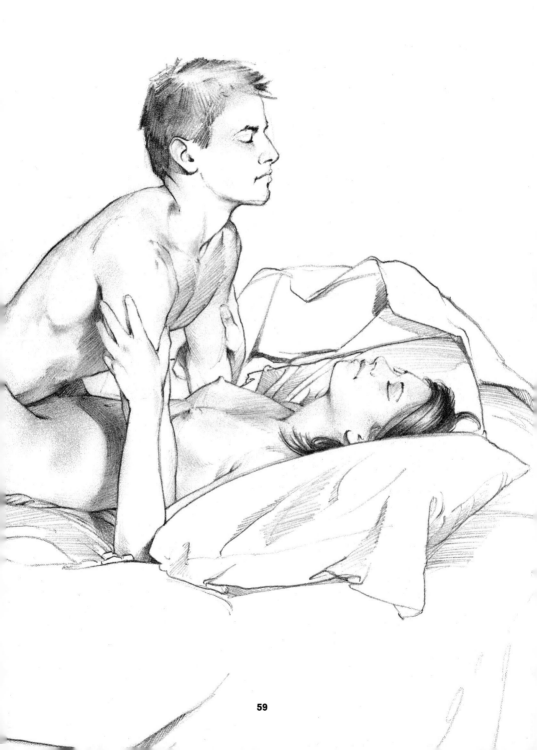

MAN ON TOP (VARIATION)

The woman can wrap her legs around your waist or neck or rest them on your shoulders. You can raise her legs by putting your forearms under her knees.

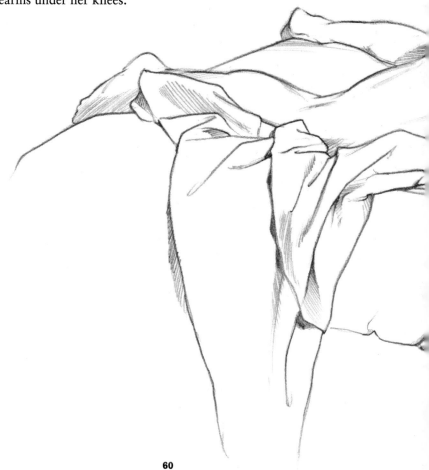

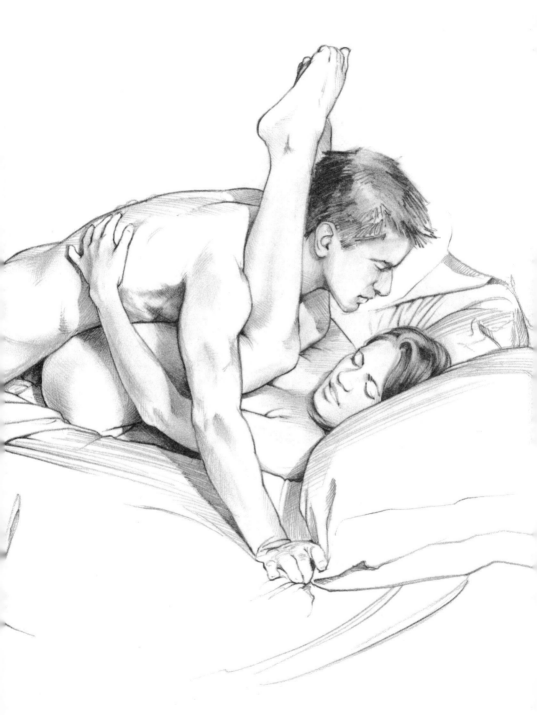

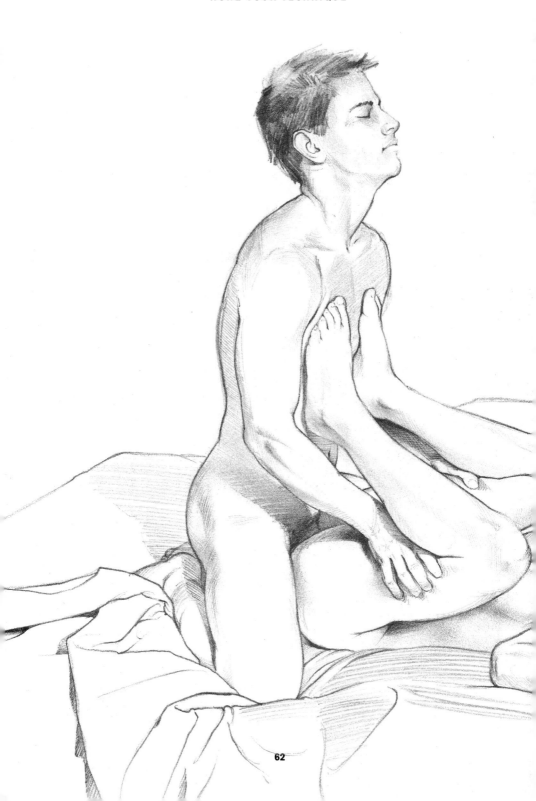

MAN ON TOP (VARIATION)

The woman can pull her knees to her chest and put her feet flat against your chest.

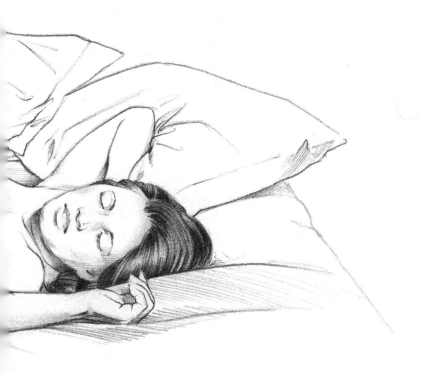

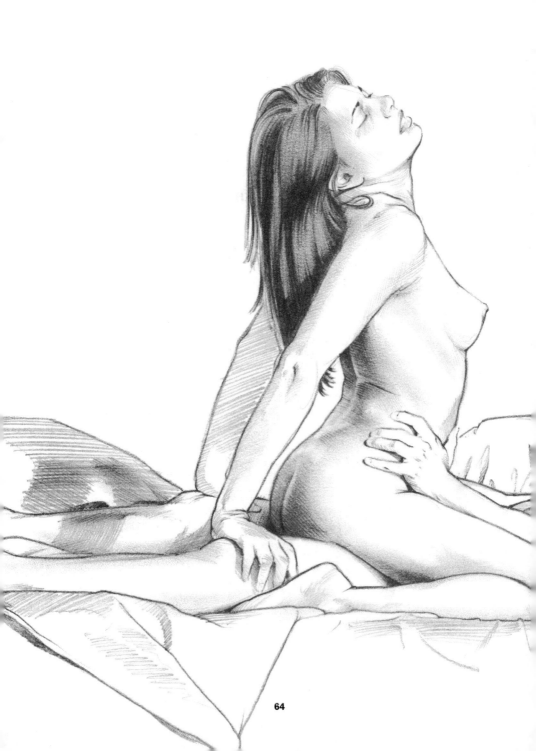

POSITION #2:WOMAN ON TOP

It's second in popularity only to the missionary position. The woman straddles your pelvis and raises and lowers herself on your penis. Like the man-on-top position, it allows you to kiss and make eye contact. The woman controls the pace as well as the angle of penetration, and she can stimulate her clitoris while you're making love.

Most men find this position visually as well as physically stimulating. You can watch your partner as she moves up and down, and your hands are free to caress her face, breasts, or buttocks. The depth of penetration equals that of the man-on-top position, which is pleasurable for both partners.

The drawbacks are the reverse of man on top. In this position, the woman rather than the man may find herself getting tired. Also, women who are self-conscious about their bodies may be somewhat uncomfortable with having them in full view.

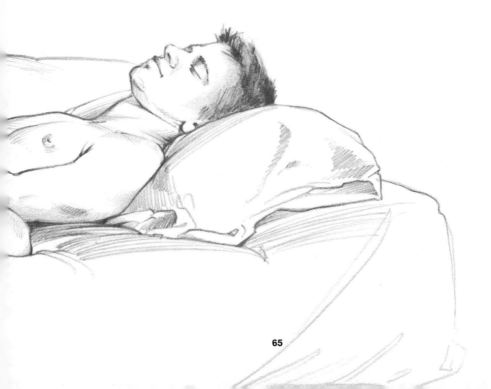

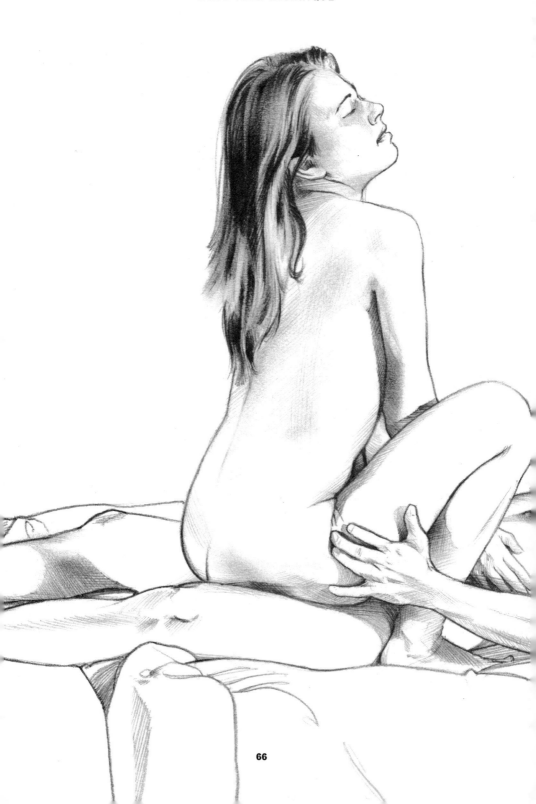

WOMAN ON TOP (VARIATION)
The woman can lean forward to rest her hands on the bed in front of her or on your chest.

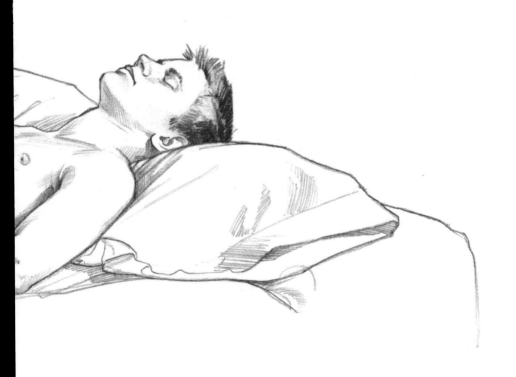

WOMAN ON TOP (VARIATION)

The woman can turn around so
she's facing your feet.

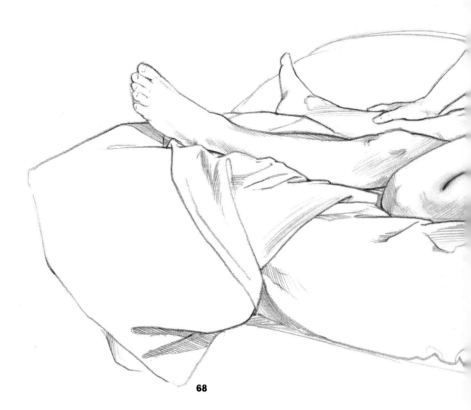

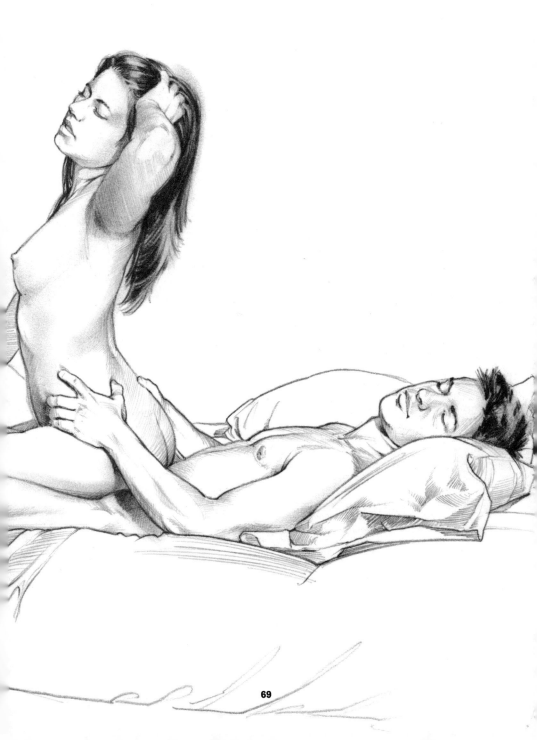

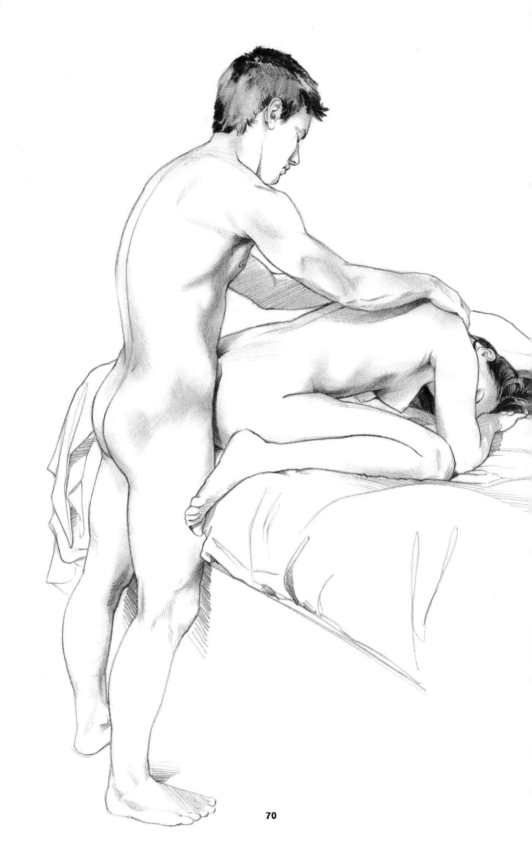

POSITION #3: REAR ENTRY

The woman gets on her knees and elbows while you enter her from behind. Many women say that this is the best position for stimulating the G-spot. It also gives her visual imagination full play; when you're out of sight, she can fill her mind with whatever fantasies she likes.

Men often enjoy this position because it gives them a sense of power and dominance, while at the same time allowing deep and vigorous thrusting. They can also reach around and touch the woman's breasts or clitoris or enjoy it while she touches herself.

The rear-entry position is less intimate than other positions, however, and some women don't like to be "taken" in the position disparagingly known as doggy style.

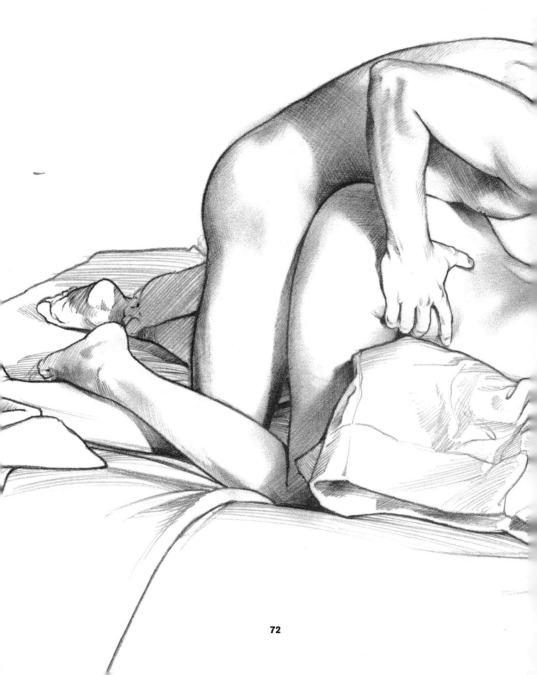

REAR ENTRY (VARIATION)

The woman can lie on her stomach with her bottom elevated.

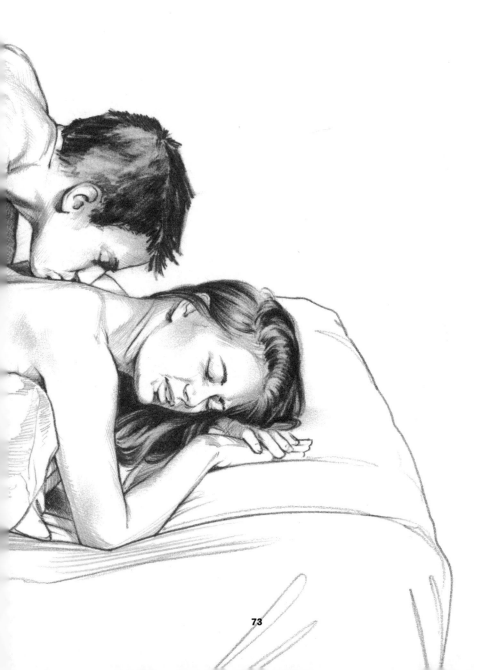

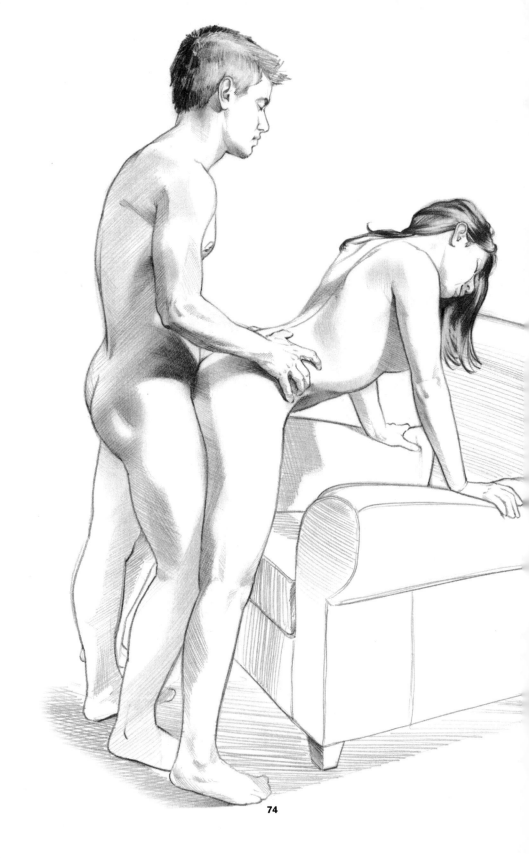

REAR ENTRY (VARIATION)

The woman can stand while bending over and holding a chair or a nightstand for support.

POSITION #4: SIDE BY SIDE

You and your partner face each other while lying on your sides. It's a good position when you're both a little tired. It's also a comfortable position if you happen to have back pain or the woman is pregnant. Side-by-side sex tends to be languorous and slow. It's easy for both partners to touch each other, and since you don't achieve deep penetration, ejaculation is often delayed.

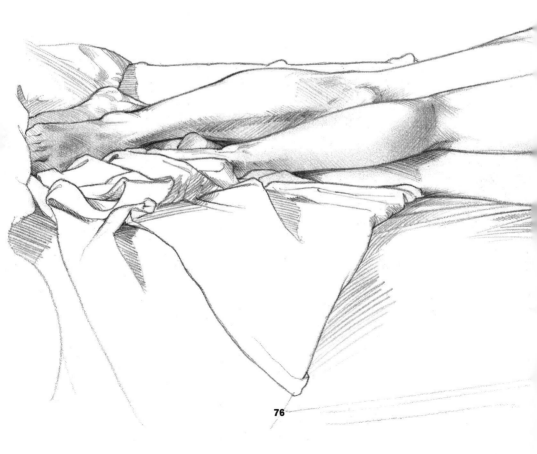

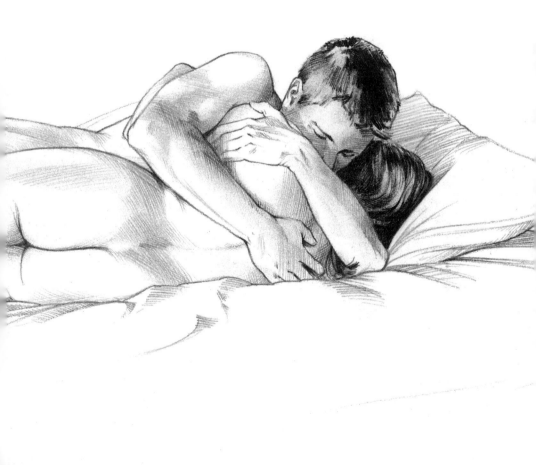

SIDE BY SIDE (VARIATION)

You can "spoon" together, with the woman's backside nestled against you.

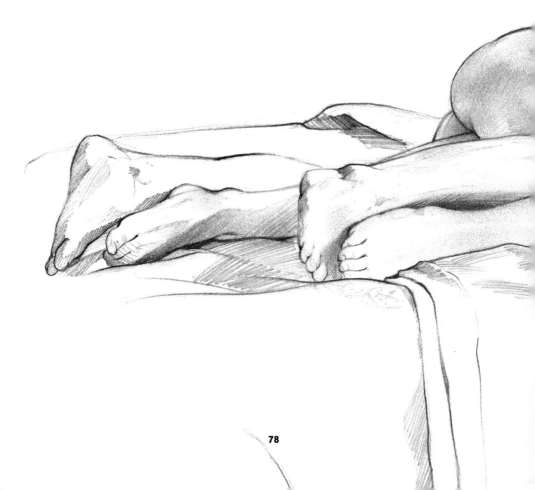

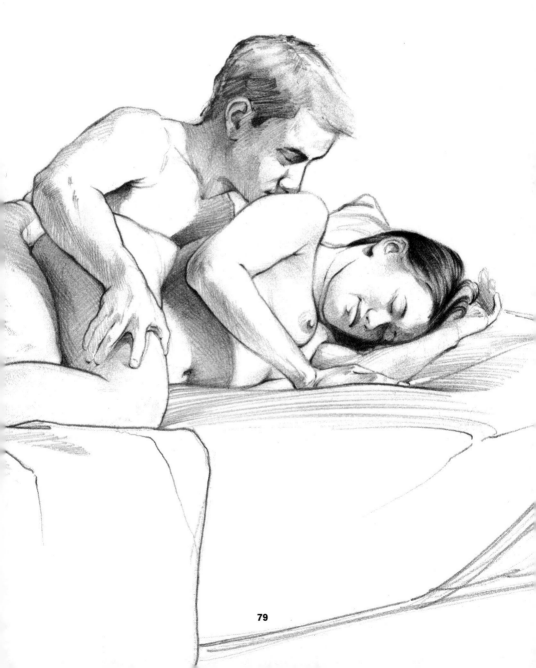

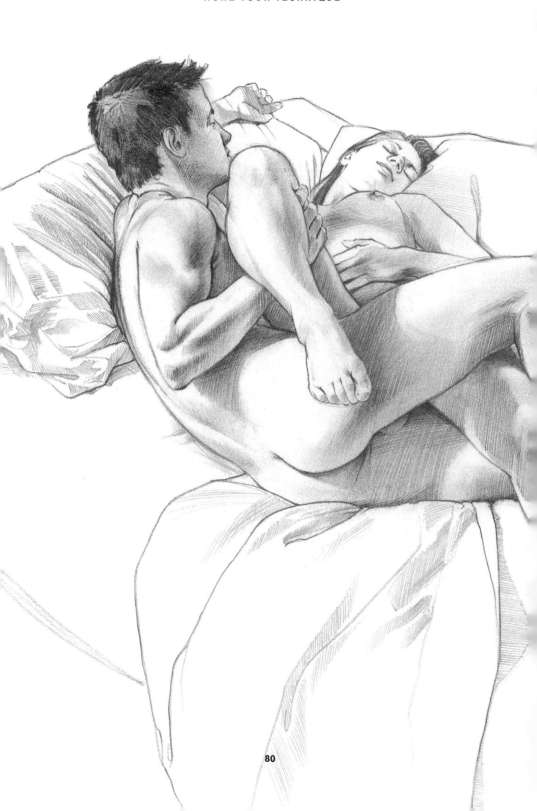

SIDE BY SIDE (VARIATION)

You can lie on your side while the woman lies on her back, one leg between your thighs and the other leg on top.

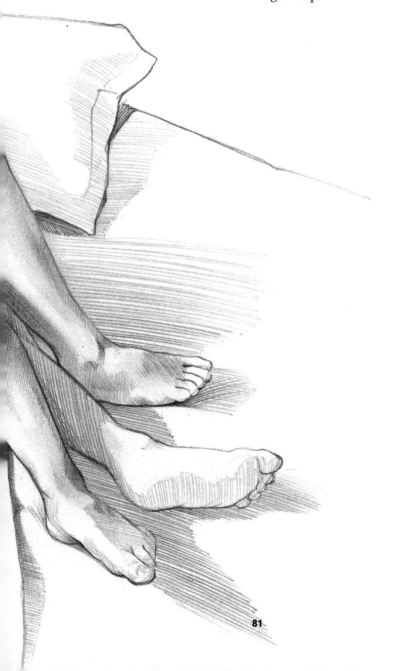

POSITION #5: SITTING

You sit on the bed while your partner sits on your lap in a face-to-face position. It's a very intimate position that permits a lot of kissing and touching. It's visually stimulating because you can fully see what your partner is doing.

Having sex while sitting is physically taxing. You have to have strong abdominal muscles to hold yourself upright. Penetration can be fairly deep, but you can't move quickly in this position.

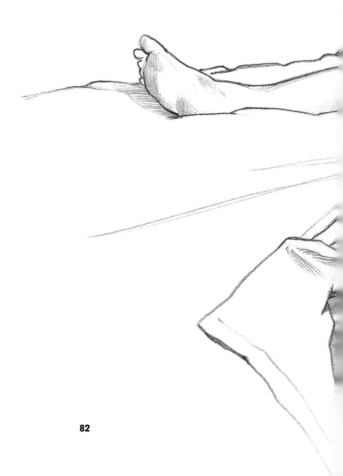

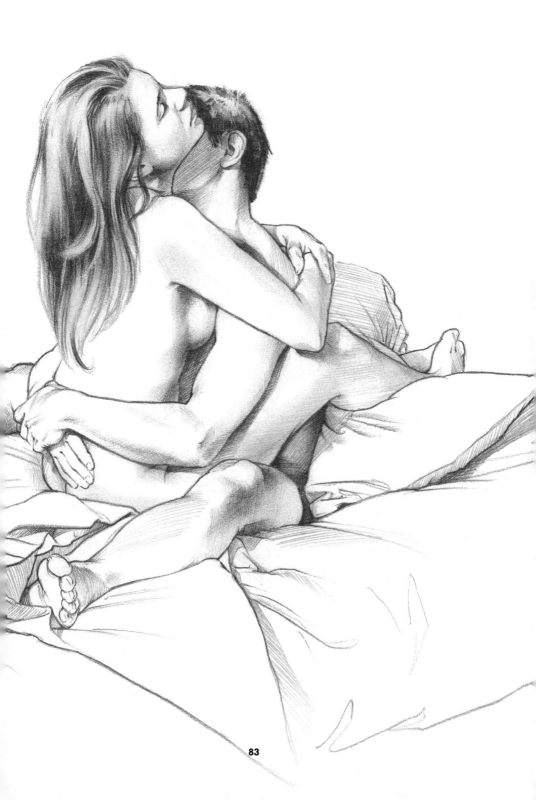

SITTING (VARIATION)

The woman can turn so that her back is against your chest.

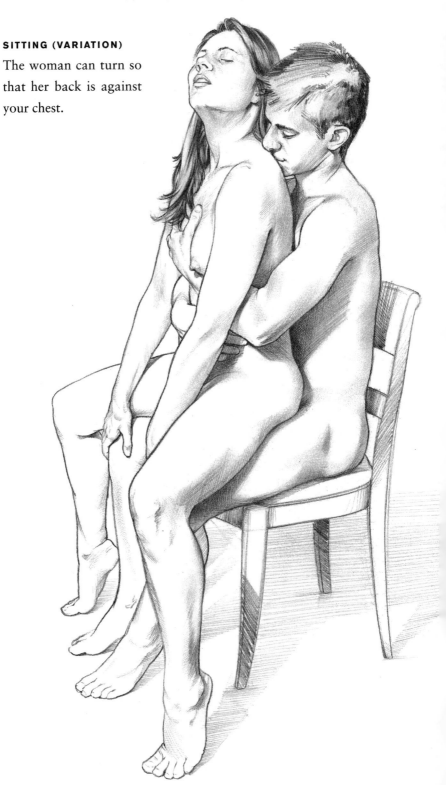

SITTING (VARIATION)

The woman can straddle you face to face in a chair, then lean all the way back to rest her head on a pillow on the floor.

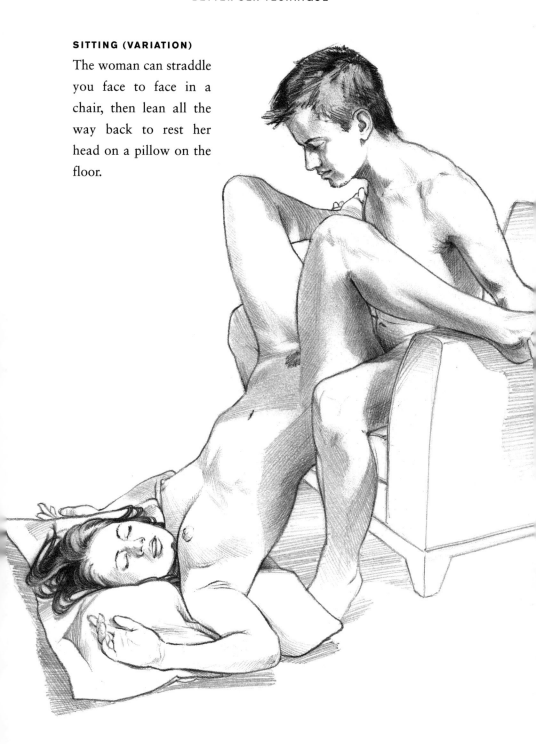

POSITION #6: STANDING

It's a good position for spontaneous lovemaking—quickies, in other words. You can enter the woman from the rear while she leans forward slightly.

This position requires more strength and dexterity than most other sexual positions. Don't try it if you have a bad back, or if your partner is too heavy to maneuver safely.

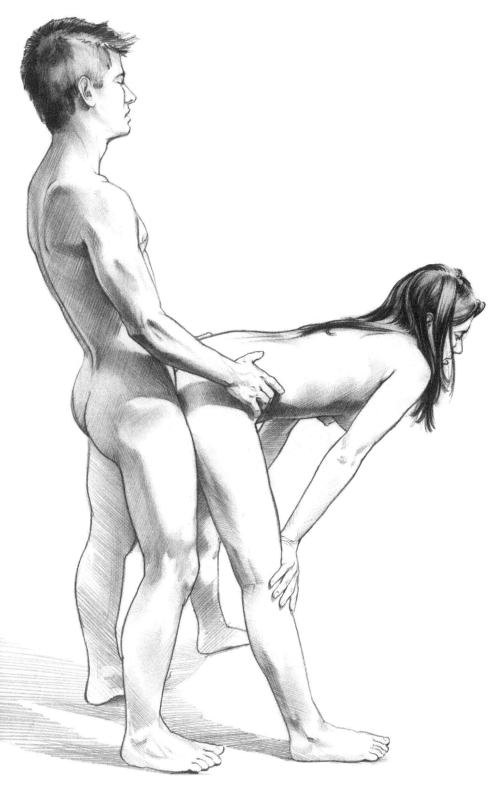

STANDING (VARIATION)

You can lift the woman with your arms, facing you, and hold her thighs while moving her up and down.

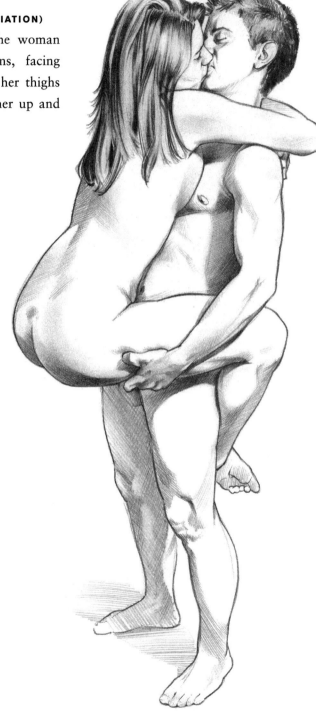

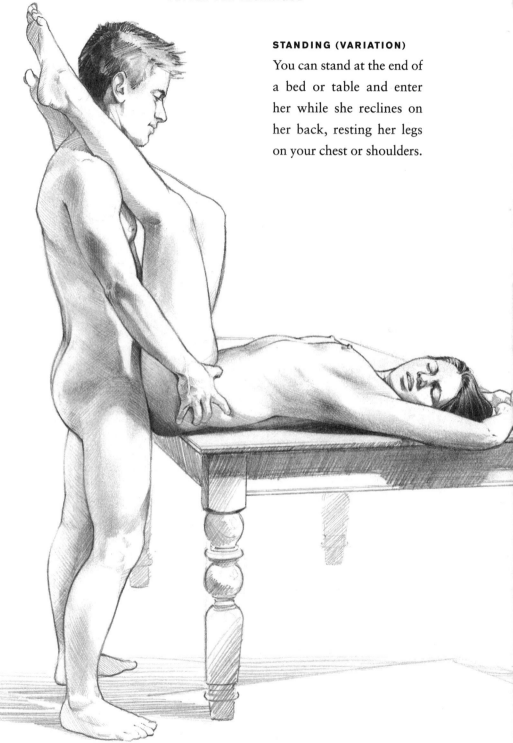

STANDING (VARIATION)

You can stand at the end of a bed or table and enter her while she reclines on her back, resting her legs on your chest or shoulders.

CREATIVE COUPLING

No matter how much you and your partner enjoy the old favorites, you might want to have some fun now and then and experiment with something totally new. It's true that there is only a handful of core positions, but each of these has almost infinite variations.

One caveat: Many of these positions take practice. If you have a mental image of porn-star dexterity and polish, you're going to be disappointed. You won't have any trouble mastering these positions, but it's going to take practice. Don't take yourself too seriously; enjoy the trying. *"Orgasms are great, but they also signal the temporary end of the fun,"* a 48-year-old firefighter told us. *"We focus more on the journey than the arrival."*

"Sex is like snow: You never know how many inches you're going to get or how long it will last."

—ANONYMOUS

▶ She lies on her back with a pillow under her butt, raises her legs high, and caresses your testicles as you enter her.

▶ She lies on her back with a pillow under her butt, legs open. You kneel between her thighs while sitting back on your ankles. Grip her thighs and pull her toward you. She can touch her clitoris while making love, and you can massage her breasts and arms.

▶ She lies on the bed or couch with her legs over the edge and her feet on the floor. You kneel and enter her without getting off your knees.

▶ Lie on your back with your legs spread at the knees. She straddles your thighs, feet resting on the bed and supporting herself with her hands, and rocks vigorously.

▶ Lie on your back with your legs apart. She straddles you, then lowers her chest to yours. She closes her thighs and clamps your penis firmly inside.

▶ Lie on your back while she straddles you. Once you're inside, sit up together and wrap your arms around each other. Sit perfectly still as your sexual energy rises. Then move gently back and forth.

▶ She lies facedown while you kneel between her legs. Pull her close and lift her buttocks for easier entry and movement.

▶ Sit on a chair while she lowers herself onto your lap, back facing you. Using her arms and legs for support, she raises and lowers herself, setting the pace and depth of penetration.

▶ She stands on a step to bring her height closer to yours, and you enter her while standing.

▶ Stand facing one another. Raise one of her legs with your hands and enter her. She supports herself with the other leg while wrapping her arms around you.

CHAPTER 4

NEXT-LEVEL TECHNIQUES

AS A MAN, YOU'RE HARDWIRED FOR SEXUAL VARIETY. AND THAT'S NOT JUST YOUR PENIS TALKING. IT'S YOUR BRAIN. Our biological bartender, Mother Nature, serves up a carnal cocktail of hormones that keeps you buzzing so you seek out sexual adventures that ultimately populate the planet.

It starts when you're single. Testosterone urges you out to bars and beaches to scout for potential mates. Once you find one, you're rewarded with a rush of amphetamine-like hormones, such as dopamine, that sends you on a hedonistic high of nonstop sex drive. You'll do it anytime, anywhere—atop the dryer, on the kitchen floor, in the garage. As time marches on with the same mate, however, that natural rush is replaced with a more mellow high from brain chemicals like vasopressin and oxytocin that calm you down enough to hold a job and raise a family. These so-called attachment chemicals leave you feeling relaxed, satisfied—and frankly, a little bored.

The key to fanning the flames is either finding a new woman (generally not an option) or pulling a fast one on Mother Nature. New positions, toys, games, and even fantasy play can make you see your partner in a whole new way—literally—by tricking your brain into responding with that feels-like-the-first-time rush. Don't take just our word for it. Women, too, need change to keep sexually charged. As a 33-year-old graphic artist from Atlanta told us. *"It's easy to get caught up in a sex routine when you've been with the same person for awhile. To keep your sex life active, you need an open mind and adventurous spirit. I enjoy being able to laugh as much as I moan (and I do both fairly loudly) during sex because we're experimenting and having fun."*

9 POSITIONS YOU DIDN'T LEARN IN SEX ED

Famed sex researcher Alfred Kinsey, Ph.D., once estimated that the missionary position was the only position used by 70 percent of the adult population. Don't tell that to the women we surveyed for this book, who unanimously rated trying new sexual positions as "very important." We flipped through ancient manuals like the *Kama Sutra* as well as some popular Web sites to bring you an arsenal of innovative, sometimes athletic, positions for sex play that should keep the fun in your bedroom for years to come.

A word to the wise: These positions may require some work (and maybe a few failed attempts) to achieve, but the payoff may be a new favorite. Says one 41-year-old Pittsburgh bartender, *"When we first started playing with new positions, it seemed more like acrobatics than sex. But a couple of times we hit upon something really, really good. That's when all the ones that didn't work out were definitely worth the effort."*

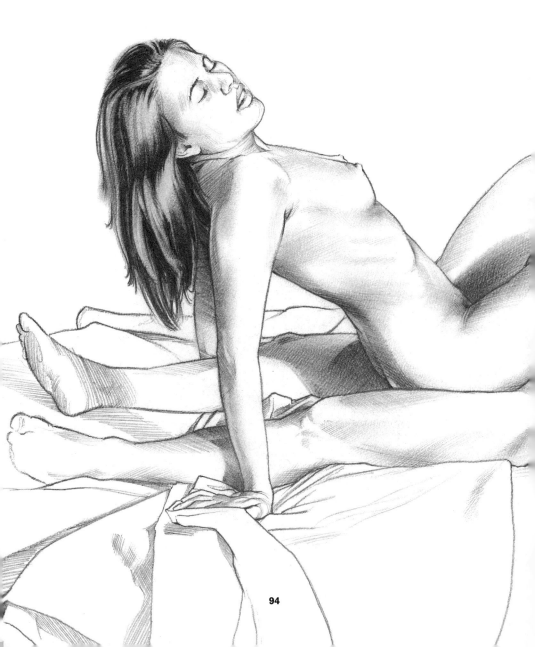

HEAD OVER HEELS

This unconventional position turns traditional sex on its head. You lie on your back with your legs slightly bent and apart. She straddles you in the classic woman-on-top position and then lies all the way back, so her feet are next to your head and her head is down by your feet. She does most of the "thrusting" by sliding back and forth along your penis.

If your penis doesn't bend that way comfortably, you can make this position more accessible by bending your knees to let her rest her back on your thighs in more of a reclining position.

Why she likes it: With her feet up by your head, you can indulge her in some decadent foot rubbing and toe sucking during intercourse.

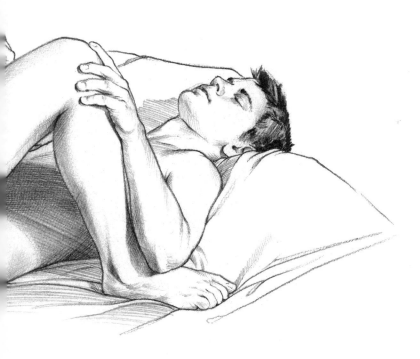

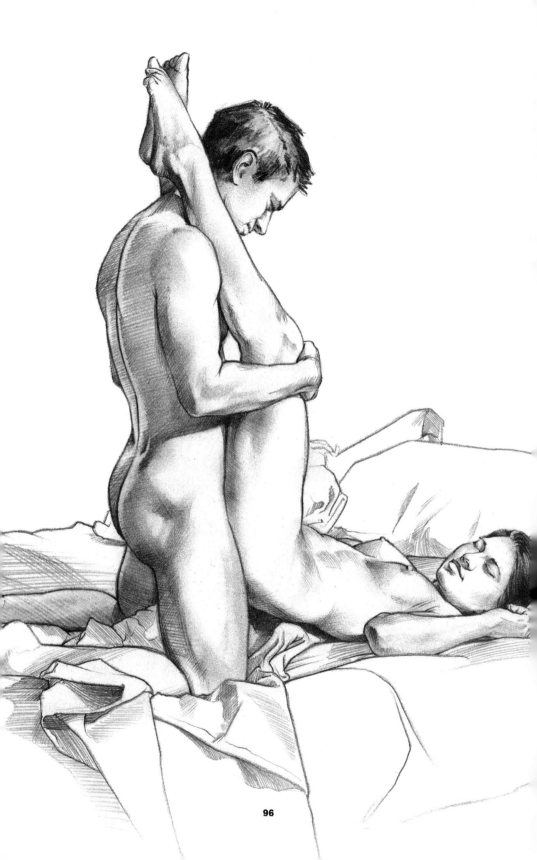

SKIN THE CAT

In this inverted position, your partner lies flat on her back; you kneel between her knees and lift her legs up and over your shoulders, so only her head and shoulders remain on the bed, and she is suspended with her calves resting on either side of your neck. You then slide your penis downward into her.

You can grasp her thighs and pull her toward you rhythmically to assist in thrusting. You also can slide your hands down and caress her clitoris for added pleasure. Though thrusting is easy from the kneeling position, men with steeply angled erections may find the downward motion of this position difficult.

Why she likes it: Being upside down gives her a giddy head rush and feeling of weightlessness during intercourse and allows her to caress her breasts.

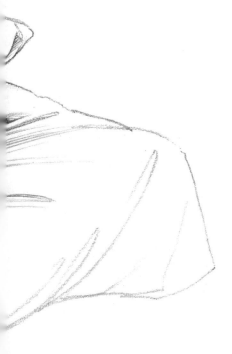

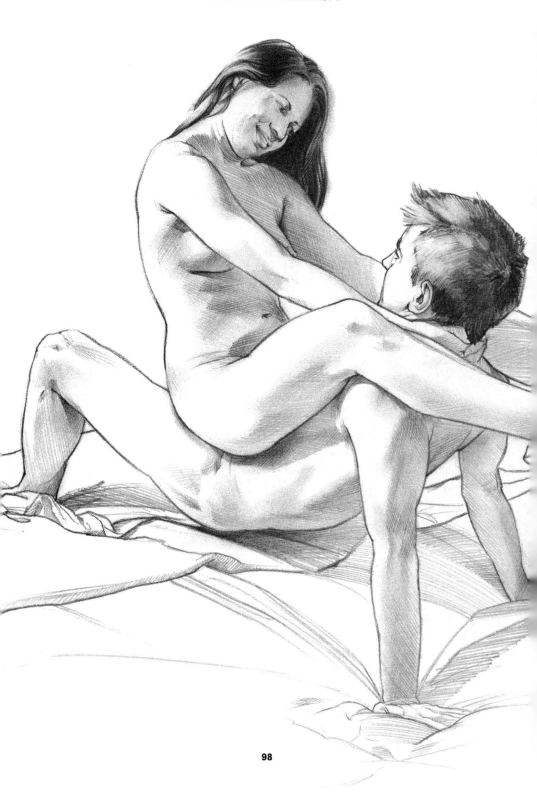

THE HONEYBEE

This part-sitting, part-reclining position allows maximum penetration and visual stimulation, though it requires a fair amount of strength and flexibility from both of you. You sit, leaning back with your hands on the bed behind your back for support. She straddles your penis, placing both legs over your shoulders and holding on to either side of your neck with her hands. To thrust, you press your thighs together, lifting her up, then open them wide, letting her slide back down, repeating so your legs make a "fluttering" motion.

The tricky part is maintaining insertion while getting into position. If she's fairly flexible, you may want to let her straddle you in the classic woman-on-top position first, then shift to place her legs over your shoulders. Otherwise, assume the position without inserting; then you can lean back and gently guide your penis into her.

Why she likes it: Her vaginal wall is angled upward, allowing for more intense G-spot stimulation with every thrust.

GAME DAY

This is a perfect position for spontaneous Sunday-afternoon sex when your favorite team is winning. You sit on a couch or cushioned armchair. She straddles you, placing her legs up and over the back or sides of the couch or chair. She can place her hands on your shoulders or place them on your knees behind her.

This position allows for a lot of variety. You can wrap your arms around each other for increased face-to-face and skin-on-skin intimacy, or she can lie all the way back and simply enjoy the ride.

Why she likes it: The seated pelvic contact here gives her extra clitoral stimulation with every thrust. Plus, you have easy access to kiss her breasts and caress her body.

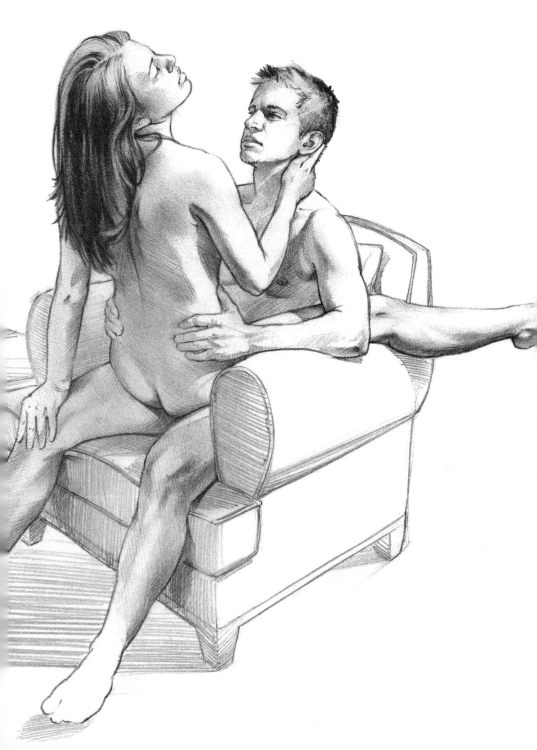

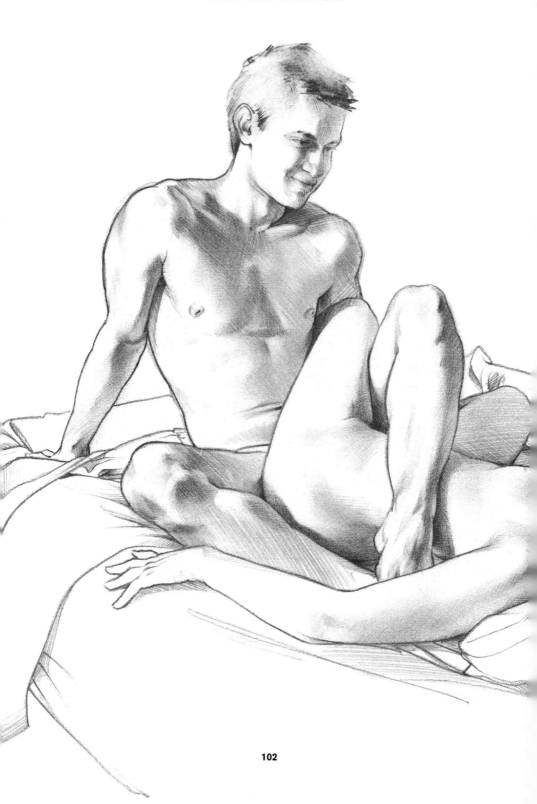

SCISSORS

Fun sex is a little like spirited grappling, and this move is reminiscent of something you might see in the WWF—only you both win. She lies back on the bed with her legs bent and thighs apart. You sit between her knees and place your right leg between her thighs so your right foot is resting by her ribs under her left arm. Grasp her left leg and bring it across your body, holding it under your left arm. Slide into her, then place your hands behind you on the bed for thrusting support. This position looks harder to achieve than it actually is, though it does require a fair amount of penile flexibility.

Why she likes it: Her clitoris will get extra stimulation as it rubs against your inner thigh during thrusting.

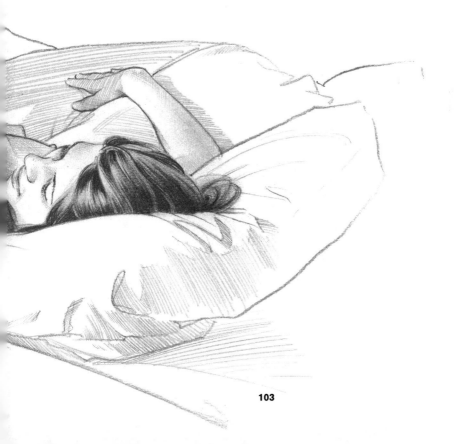

BLUE MOON

Like all good positions, this one begins sexy and gets hotter as it progresses. To begin, you lie face up on the bed as usual. She straddles you facing your feet. Once your penis is fully inserted, she bends all the way forward, so her breasts are resting on your thighs and her face is down by your shins. She also can extend her legs slightly to fully drape herself over you as you thrust in unison.

Why she likes it: She can rub her breasts against your legs. And you can increase her pleasure by rubbing her buttocks and caressing her labia as you slide in and out of her.

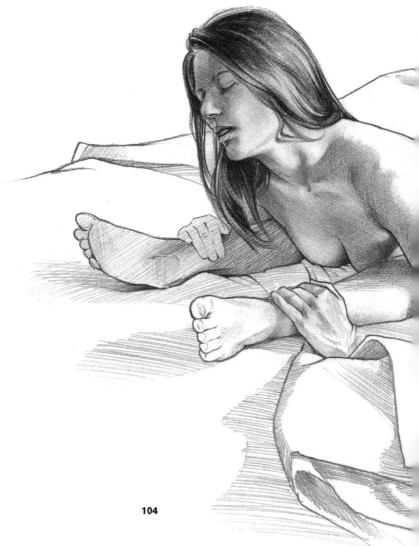

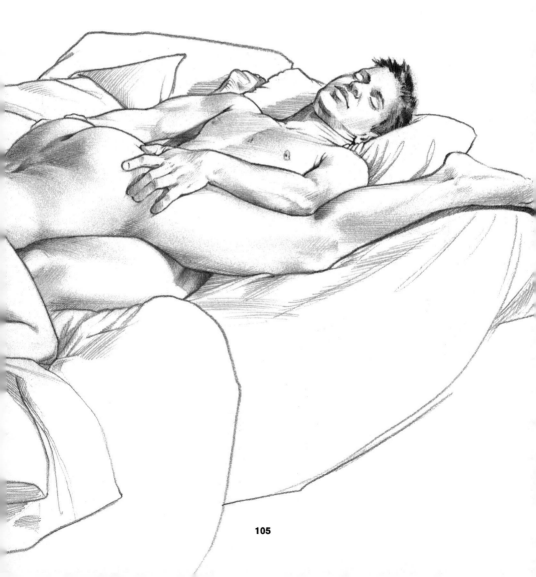

ON BENDED KNEE

In this erotic take on the classic marriage proposal pose, you kneel on the bed, and she kneels down in front of you with her right leg bent so it drapes over your left leg and the lower part of her left leg extended behind her for balance and support. Hold onto her hips and enter her, thrusting as you normally would.

If she is a lot shorter than you, she may need to kneel on pillows to achieve this position.

Why she likes it: This position has romantic undertones and allows for lots of face-to-face intimacy, kissing, and caressing.

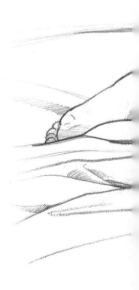

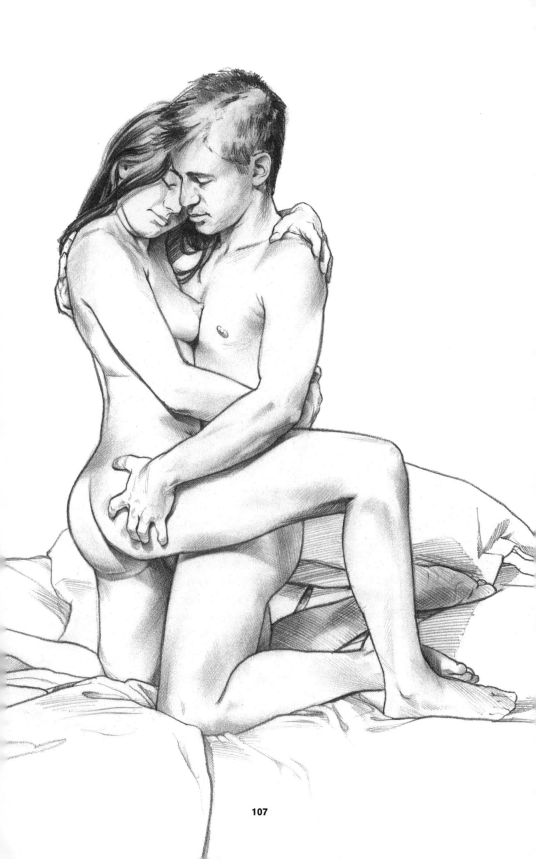

THE WHEELBARROW

As the name implies, this position harkens back to the childhood game where you pick up someone's legs as if using a wheelbarrow. Only now it's a lot more fun. Have your partner lie facedown on a carpeted floor. Step between her feet, grasp her legs, and lift her lower body off the floor. As you lift, she should straighten her arms and support herself on her hands, so you can lift her vagina to you and slide your penis into her from behind.

Why she likes it: This variation of the rear-entry position tilts her pelvis so she feels more G-spot stimulation with every thrust.

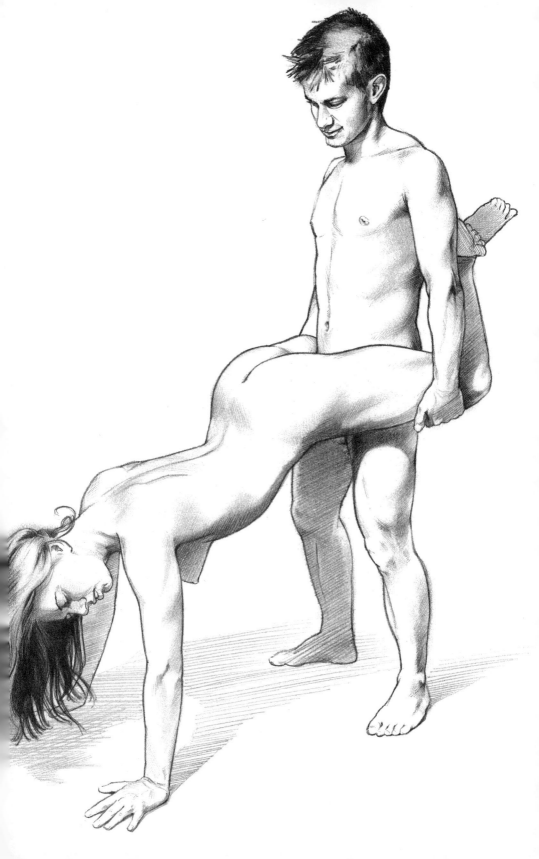

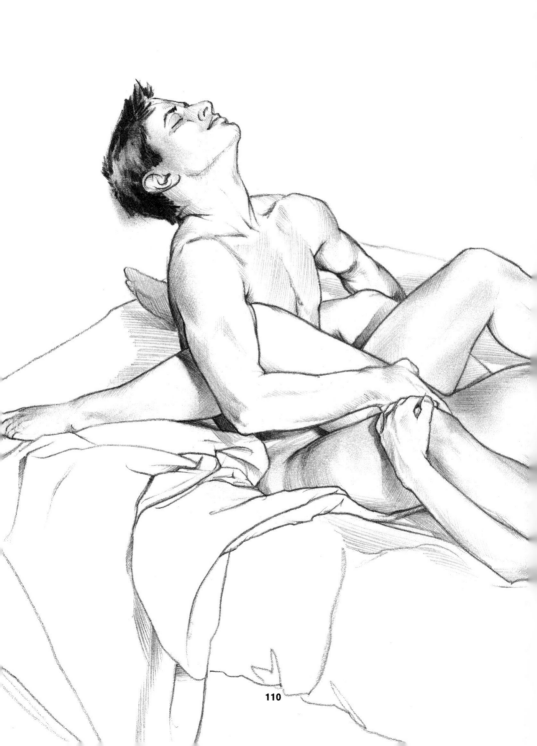

THE PRETZEL

In this twisty-turny position, you recline with your right leg extended and your left leg bent. Your thighs should be apart and your torso should be off the bed about 45 degrees. She lies between your legs with her head on the bed by your right foot, weaving her right leg under your left and draping her left leg over your right as you enter her. She wraps her left arm around your right thigh, and you hold onto her waist for thrusting leverage.

Why she likes it: This pretzel position gives her easy access to massage her clitoris at a pressure she enjoys while fully reclined and comfortable.

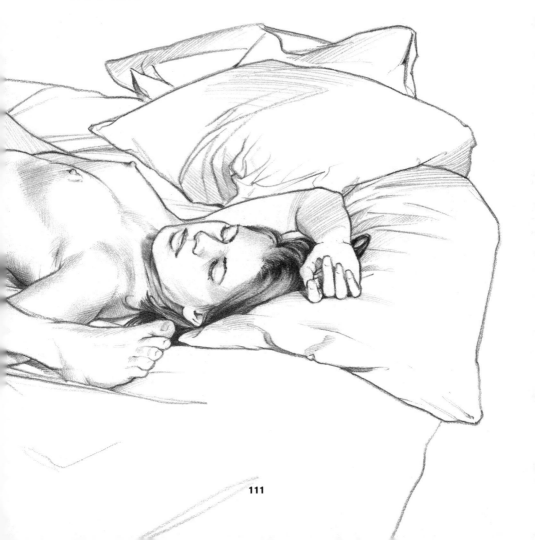

TOYS FOR TWO

Sexual aids have been used around the globe for more than a thousand years. Back in the day, they were mostly considered male-replacement apparatus. The Greek *olisbos* and Italian *diletto* were designed to give solace to lonely women whose husbands were out fighting or foraging. In the Victorian era, doctors actually invented the first vibrator, used to treat "female hysteria," literally "suffering of the uterus." Today, toys are used as much, if not more, for couple fun as for solitary pleasure—and vibrators seem to be the toy of choice. *"A vibrator is a fun way to mix things up during sex,"* says a 38-year-old software engineer from Eatontown, New Jersey. *"It also helps me know my body better, which is helpful for both of us."* Some women especially like to use their toys on their partners. Said one 44-year-old nurse from Jacksonville, Florida, *"Sex toys make it easier to see how your handiwork is pleasing your partner. That's a big turn on."*

The take-home lesson: If you're interested, talk to your partner. Surf women-friendly Web sites like www.goodvibes.com or www.babeland.com and pick out a toy for each of you. Here's a primer to get you started.

VIBRATORS. These popular toys come in all shapes and sizes. Some lifelike. Some shaped like rabbits or toy soldiers. Some insertable. Some not. Many are designed for stimulating specific areas—the clitoris or G-spot, for example, or both at the same time. Some even feature special devices for simultaneous clitoral, G-spot, and anal stimulation. Vibrators range in price from $8 to $80.

Your main choice when selecting a vibrator is whether it should plug in or be battery operated. The best-selling model year after year at Good Vibrations in San Francisco is the Hitachi Magic Wand, a long-handled electric vibrator with a soft round head. It is also available in a rechargeable model, so you can enjoy it without getting tangled up in wires.

CLEAN AND HEALTHY

Using a dildo or vibrator is a good safe-sex option. Just make sure you wash it thoroughly or put a condom on it before transferring it from the anus to the vagina or mouth. Better yet, put a condom on it any time you use it. The same advice goes for using a finger or your penis in the anal area: Don't put it in other orifices without washing it thoroughly first or changing the condom. The anus hosts bacteria that can cause infections elsewhere.

Battery-operated vibrators are less expensive and generally more portable, though they are less durable and powerful. If your partner likes a good buzz, you also can treat her to a hands-free vibrator, which fits snugly against her clitoris with a jockstrap-like harness. The newest version, the Audi-Oh, is activated by sound. You can plug it into your stereo to let her groove to the music, or you can sweet-talk her into bliss Barry White–style. Hands-free vibrators also can be worn during intercourse. That way, you can enjoy the vibrations, too.

DILDOS. Taking their name from the Italian *diletto,* meaning "delight," these toys are designed for insertion. They range in size from pinkie-finger small to overgrown-zucchini large. Though most are shaped like the real deal, they also come in nonanatomical shapes like a whale or dolphin. Some vibrate and have extra protrusions for clitoral and/or anal stimulation. You can buy a simple rubber dildo for about $15, but for top quality, go with a silicone model (prices average about $30 to $40). They're easier to clean, and, unlike cold rubber, silicone retains body heat and feels better during play.

ANAL PLUGS. These smaller members of the dildo family are expressly designed for anal stimulation, which both you and your partner can enjoy either during intercourse or solo. What makes anal plugs special is that they have a flared base to prevent them from getting caught in the rectum. Start with the smallest one you can find and work your way to a larger size over time. Insert the toy gently, using liberal amounts of lubrication to avoid tearing delicate anal and rectal tissue. Let the toy just sit there at first, responding to normal body movement. After a while, when the sensation becomes comfortable, try gently moving it in and out. Anal plugs cost about $15.

BALLS AND BEADS. Ben wa balls have been enjoyed in Asian countries for more than a thousand years. These golf ball–size toys are hollow and contain another ball inside, which provides a pleasant "thumping" sensation as they bump against one another inside a woman's vagina. For anal stimulation, try anal beads— marble-size silicone beads threaded together on a string and secured in place with a silicone ring. They can be inserted before intercourse or oral sex, then gently pulled out one at a time for intense stimulation during orgasm. Balls and beads range in price from $5 to $25.

RINGS AND SLEEVES. Though most sex toys are created for women, these you can call your own. Most notable in this category is the constriction device, or cock ring. By placing the ring at the base of your erection, you trap blood in the erectile chamber and stay hard longer. Though these toys can enhance your pleasure, don't get carried away with them. Constrictor rings cut off fresh blood flow to your penis and should never be worn longer than 20 minutes, or you risk serious tissue damage. To avoid injury, get one that is made of soft leather or latex and adjustable with Velcro, snaps, or a bolo tie.

"Sleeves" slide over the penis to provide a snug, warm, moist sensation (like the real thing) during manual stimulation. Some even vibrate. Rings and sleeves run about $5 to $20.

LUBRICANTS. Designed to make caressing and insertion more sensuous and slippery, lubricants can be used with sex toys or by themselves during intercourse and massage. The women we spoke to love their lubes. *"Lubricants cut down on friction and soreness after a lo-o-ong, fun time,"* explained a 25-year-old Denver graduate student. *"The commercial varieties are almost better than what nature has provided,"* confessed a 33-year-old paralegal from St. Louis. They come in a wide variety, too. You'll find body rubs in every flavor and scent. There are even special heating oils that warm up when you blow on them. At just $3 a pop, they're a cheap, easy way to spice up everyday sex.

GAMES. If your partner is a little shy about sexual experimentation, a sex game can be a great way to break the ice. Designed with women in mind, board and dice games are short on rules and shorter on competition, offering gentle ways to coax her into being sexually adventurous. Most board games just ask you to do little erotic things that seem silly but encourage communication, along with arousal. For example, a card may tell you, "Touch your partner somewhere you've never touched before." Or you may land on a space and be instructed to spread whipped cream on your body where you'd like your partner to lick it off.

BACKDOOR PLAY

According to a *Redbook* study of 100,000 women, 43 percent of women have tried anal sex with their partners at least once. Not surprisingly, about half did not enjoy it. Forty percent reported finding pleasure in this still stigmatized sex act, and the remaining women gave it neither yay nor nay.

Though anal sex sounds difficult and uncomfortable, if not painful, it *does* have the potential to be quite enjoyable. That's because the lining of the anal cavity is brimming with feel-good nerve endings that add pleasure to foreplay and intercourse when stimulated. For the man, the tightness of the anus can provide a new, powerful sensation during intercourse.

Facts and stats aside, don't be surprised if your partner puts the kibosh on backdoor exploration. If you're curious, approach the subject—and the act—carefully and gently. If she doesn't react with a straight-armed forget-about-it, chances are she's game to try, if just once. One woman who told us she enjoyed anal stimulation offered this advice, "*Go slow! A glass of wine helps everyone relax. Lots of good lubricant is a must. Using a very small dildo first can help. If she says 'no more' at any time, stop immediately.*" Other tips:

START CLEAN. Showering or bathing together before anal sex will help you both get as clean as possible inside and out.

SCORE A HAT TRICK

Most of us rely on the clitoris like the automatic garage door opener. It's a go-to button to gain rumbling access when we want to park our car. But there's more to the female orgasm than massage, rub, repeat. Though clitoral stimulation provides a reliable orgasm, your partner may experience intense, multiple, simultaneous orgasms if you stimulate two—or three—of her hot spots at the same time.

Next time you're manually or orally stimulating your partner's clitoris, insert a finger in her vagina and locate the rough, raised G-spot on the front of her vaginal wall. Stimulate both with about equal pressure until she comes to a shuddering "bigasm"—an orgasm that comes from both erogenous zones.

Then take it to the next level. Following the same directions as above, use your other hand to reach under her and gently stimulate her anal area with your fingertips. The resulting "trigasm" will deliver a high-voltage, full-body release. With some maneuvering, you can achieve the same result during intercourse. In the woman-on-top position, have her tilt her hips forward so that your penis hits her G-spot and her clitoris is rubbing against your shaft with every thrust. Then reach around and simultaneously stimulate her anal area with your fingertips.

ASK FIRST. Never just wander a finger or your penis to that general area and start poking around. That's likely to elicit a clamp-down.

PROTECT YOURSELF. Even if you and your partner have been together since the dinosaurs and are 100 percent disease free, you should wear a condom during anal sex to prevent getting an infection from the bacteria in the rectum. A well-lubricated condom will also be easier on her during insertion.

LUBRICATE LIBERALLY. The rectum is not a self-lubricating area like the vagina. It is also *much* more susceptible to painful tearing. Apply a water-based lubricant like K-Y Jelly to yourself and to her before you start. Add more as needed.

USE SUPER SLOW-MO. She must be completely relaxed and receptive if there is any hope for successful anal sex. That means taking your time. Start with your pinkie finger or a small dildo. Work up to just the tip of your penis. Once inside, ease in as slowly as possible or let her bear down on you. If she says enough, stop then and there. If she wants out, pull out. Once you get to the point of thrusting, do so slowly and very, very gently.

TIE ME UP, TIE ME DOWN

Power-play sex has gotten a bad rap in popular entertainment. In Stephen King's *Gerald's Game,* a woman is left cuffed in a remote cabin after her kink-loving hubby bites it during rough sex. In *Basic Instinct,* the tables turn, and it's the men who take it to heart (literally) with an ice pick while submitting to a little tie-and-tease action. But the truth is, plenty of perfectly normal, nonhomicidal couples enjoy a little playful bondage and discipline (B&D) now and then.

"Bondage of any kind requires a lot of trust. If that trust is there, not being able to see what's coming next can be very exciting," says a 44-year-old medical worker from suburban Philadelphia. *"Tell her*

exactly what you are going to do, step by step (no pain, please, unless she's into it). The anticipation will get her so wet you can forget about lubes." The key word here, though, is *trust.* A surprising number of women we talked to, even happily married ones who gleefully dallied with dildos and anal play, took a step back at the suggestion of being tied up. More than a few said simply, *"I'm not trusting enough."*

Because bondage and discipline treads into sensitive areas of power and control, it's not only essential that you get your partner's consent, it may be necessary for you to show your trust by giving her the ties first. She will likely be more comfortable and willing to play along when she has the pleasure of calling the initial shots.

Before you embark on any B&D adventure, agree on a code word that means "Stop now. I've had enough." Having such a signal (called a safeword in bondage lingo) leaves you free to scream and beg and bully as much as you want to as part of the fun, knowing that the one and only safeword will put an end to things if they get too rough or one of you starts feeling uncomfortable.

Some people like to throw a little sadomasochism (S&M) into the mix. Many women (and men) enjoy gentle spanking and nipple squeezing during foreplay and intercourse. But don't pull out the leather riding crop unless you've talked it over ahead of time. Any unpleasant surprises can result in a big sexual setback.

The sexually adventurous can buy elaborate handcuffs, blindfolds, and harnesses for all this naughty play. But homemade restraints (silk scarves, neckties) work just as well and don't need to be hidden from friends and family.

FANTASY IN REALITY

You were just there to mow the lawn, maybe plant a few petunias, and there she was, the hot, horny housewife lying by the pool, wearing nothing but a silk scarf and a come-and-get-me smile. Her husband could come home at any minute, but who can resist 10 minutes of afternoon delight? After you're done, you can be a hardened criminal, and she'll be the warden. Or a pilot and a flight attendant. Therein lies the beauty of fantasy—it gives your subconscious a chance to play games limited only by your imagination.

Experts have different theories on the origin of sexual fantasy. Some say it's our brains playing out desires we've accumulated since birth. Others argue that sexual daydreams are a survival mechanism of sorts—a way of playing out situations that could be immoral, dangerous, or illegal. The one point they all agree on: We all have them, and we should simply enjoy them rather than reading too much into what it all means.

One way to enjoy this mental sexual theater is to do what we all already do—use them as fodder for masturbation. It also can be fun to bring them to life in a safe way by role playing with your partner. The biggest barrier here is embarrassment. Many women feel awkward or just plain stupid dressed up as French maids. But if you can help your partner through her inhibitions, often by taking the first step yourself, she may be willing to play along.

One cautionary note: When sharing your fantasies, use common sense. You may regard your interest in riding reverse cowgirl with the local lifeguard as an innocent diversion of the mind, but she may mistake it as an actual desire to stray. Communicate, play it smart, and keep your fantasy exploits anonymous. Or better yet, let her take center stage in your most erotic theatrics. Some popular fantasies to play out:

FOOTBALL PLAYER AND HEAD CHEERLEADER. Lift her skirt and go for a score.

BUSINESS EXECUTIVE AND SEXY INTERN. Call a private meeting and ask her to take some very personal dictation.

TEACHER AND STUDENT. She's Mrs. Robinson, and you're a very bad boy.

NURSE AND PATIENT. A kiss and caress for wherever it hurts.

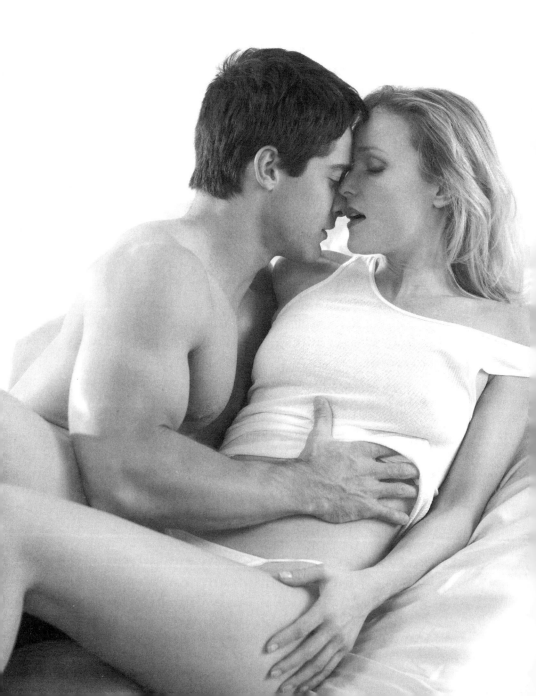

PART 2

MAXIMIZE
PLEASURE
CONTROL

CHAPTER 5

HARDER, LONGER

HOW LONG DOES IT TAKE YOU TO COME DURING SEX? IF YOU'RE LIKE MOST MEN, YOU PROBABLY CLOCK IN AT AROUND 3 MINUTES. That's fine for a quickie, but not necessarily long enough for over-the-top enjoyment—yours as well as hers. How about your erections? Are they hard enough for satisfying sex? Again, the average man has some issues in this area. Between 20 and 30 million American men can't perform the way they'd like, and we *all* have trouble from time to time.

Obviously, every man responds differently to erotic stimulation, and context always makes a difference: your mood, how much you've had to drink, the quality of your relationship with your partner, and so on. Some men ejaculate almost immediately after starting sex, and if they've had good foreplay and are in a comfortable relationship, they might be perfectly happy with their performance. Another man might last 5, 10, or 20 minutes and be disappointed that he came so quickly.

There's so much individual variation in sexual expectations and performance that it's a stretch to call anything normal. But we know in our guts that we're supposed to perform in certain ways, and we feel a sting of disappointment when we don't. Worse, the penis—and by extension, a man's perception of his sexual performance—is often the butt of lame jokes in a way that a woman's genitals or performance aren't. We might laugh when someone makes a joke about a "pencil dick" or being too "quick on the trigger," but behind the laughter, there's a lot of sexual anxiety.

Curiously, it's men themselves who create much of the stress. Women, numerous surveys show, are relatively unconcerned about the size of a man's penis, how long he lasts, or whether he's always hard and ready.

"We have anxiety of our own about our bodies being judged and whether or not we'll be able to have an orgasm," says a 29-year-old marine biologist in Galveston, Texas, who responded to our survey. *"Men should relax and know that getting there is just as much fun."*

Indeed, men who learn how to relax, who accept the fact that their bodies aren't machines that can be programmed to perform on command, generally have fewer problems with erections or too-early ejaculation than those who work themselves up into sweaty knots of anxiety. In addition, every man can learn to improve just about every parameter of sexual performance, such as the frequency and duration of erections, how hard erections get, and how long he lasts during sex. An obvious point, one that we frequently overlook, is that the penis *is* a machine of sorts, just as your muscles are machines, and can be improved with specific exercises.

The vast majority of men don't need a whole lot of work to kick their sexual performance up a notch or two. We're talking a couple of minutes a day at most—and as you'll see, they'll be some of the most pleasurable minutes you've ever experienced.

ANATOMY OF AN ERECTION

The penis carries way too much emotional baggage, especially when you consider that on the purely physical level, it's mainly a conduit for urine and semen and is made up largely of nerves, muscles, and blood.

Let's start with the issue of size. The average man has about 6 inches of *visible* penis. The other half is rooted deep inside the body, extending nearly back to the anus. The "root" of the penis, which ducks under the prostate gland, forks into two branches that attach to the pelvic bone, which holds the whole thing in place.

INSIDE THE PENIS

The penis is more than 50 percent muscle, and a hefty percentage of that muscle is found in the tiny blood vessels that lace through it like lines on a road map. It's no accident that the penis is blood-rich terrain. When you're sexually aroused, signals from the brain (or

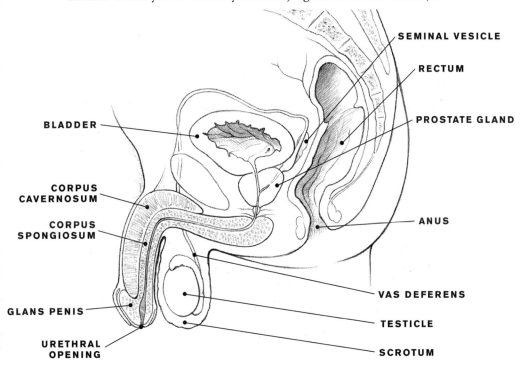

SEMINAL VESICLE

RECTUM

PROSTATE GLAND

BLADDER

CORPUS CAVERNOSUM

CORPUS SPONGIOSUM

ANUS

VAS DEFERENS

GLANS PENIS

TESTICLE

URETHRAL OPENING

SCROTUM

from the penis itself) tell blood vessels to relax. Blood flows through the tissues and gets temporarily locked in place, causing an erection.

Let's say you're spending a quiet night at home watching TV. Your thumb, apparently with a mind of its own, clicks to a cable channel featuring a little adult entertainment. The movie is hot, and your brain responds by sending stimuli down neural pathways all the way to your penis. Blood pours into the corpora cavernosa, the tubes of tissue that constitute the core of the penis. Within minutes or less, the amount of blood in the penis can increase by a factor of 10. At the same time, the expanding penile tissues squeeze against blood vessel walls and prevent blood from getting out. If you're generally healthy, you're probably pretty hard at this point—and will stay that way until the sexy nerve transmissions stop.

Nature takes erections seriously. To make sure they occur, there are two separate nerve pathways to the penis. The first comes into

"BLUE BALLS": FACT OR FANCY?

Generations of eager men have tried to shame generations of reluctant women into having sex by playing victim politics: "Honey, we have to have sex right now to get rid of this *agonizing* pain."

There is a kernel of truth to these protestations of pain, but just barely. When a man is sexually aroused, blood flows into the penis and testicles, then just as quickly flows out when he comes. However, blood leaves the scene more slowly when he doesn't ejaculate. The pressure from accumulated blood can in fact make the testicles a little achy.

However, the discomfort rarely lasts longer than a few minutes, and it's hardly agonizing. A guy who truly feels uncomfortable can always go home and take care of things himself. In most cases, though, he doesn't need relief at all, just a little patience. Insisting makes for lousy sex—and worse relationships.

play when, say, you or your partner strokes your penis. An erection can occur pretty much automatically, whether or not you're thinking sexy thoughts. It's just a basic reflex. The second pathway travels directly from the brain and is triggered by erotic thoughts—the kind generated by the aforementioned adult movie, for example.

The best erections, those that are hardest and feel best, usually involve signals from *both* nervous pathways working in delightful harmony.

MORE BLOOD, MORE PLEASURE

Okay, so you need blood, a lot of it, to get and maintain a good erection. A lot of men, especially those 40 and older, simply don't get enough. Psychological factors such as stress or performance anxiety can certainly cause problems, but they aren't the main culprits. Doctors estimate that about 70 percent of men who suffer frequent erection problems have an underlying vascular problem or diseases that affect nerves as well as bloodflow, such as diabetes.

No man wants to discuss sexual problems with anyone, including doctors. Do it anyway. For one thing, the vast majority of men who aren't performing the way they'd like can improve dramatically with medical treatment, counseling, or a combination of both. Why suffer in bed if you don't have to? More important, some of the same conditions that restrict bloodflow to the penis can also impede circulation to other parts of the body, such as the heart. You've got to find out what's going on, or you could find yourself with more to worry about than an erection—like a heart attack.

Since the focus of this chapter is on ways to make erections (and orgasms) better and more reliable, this isn't the place to dwell on the many causes and treatments of full-fledged erection problems. (We discuss these problems at length in chapters 12 and 13.) That said, almost any man will notice an improvement in sexual vigor if he does a few simple things.

WHACK THE WINGS. The usual nutritional advice is about as interesting as front-row seats at the World Shuffleboard Invitational. But there's a good reason that doctors almost beg guys to eat at least five daily servings of vegetables, along with plenty of fruit—and to cut back on the buffalo wings and Krispy Kremes. The more fat and cholesterol you have sloshing around in your blood, the more likely you are to wake up one day with thick, sticky deposits on the walls of your arteries. The blood vessels that you need for erections are a lot smaller than the pipes leading to the heart. Even a small amount of sludge can cause a lot of sexual embarrassment.

▼

Men of the French Renaissance aristocracy thought that they could increase penis size by hanging money bags from their erections. They'd keep adding gold coins or jewels until the bag slid off. They believed that the penis had reached its optimal size when the bag stayed in place for 2 minutes.

▲

GIVE UP THE SMOKES. Not "someday"—now. Smoking vastly increases the rate of atherosclerosis, nature's equivalent of blood vessel cement. The equation, remember, boils down to this: Bad bloodflow = bad erections.

CHECK YOUR MEDS. Dozens of prescription drugs can take the heat out of your sexual furnace. If you're having erection problems and are taking antidepressants, tranquilizers, appetite suppressants, or ulcer drugs such as Tagamet (cimetidine), have a chat with your doc. Switching to a different drug will probably deliver the same benefits without the sexual downside.

LOG SOME COUCH TIME. Yes, it's uncomfortable at first to discuss intimate problems with a therapist, and yes, it can be expensive, but there's a reason that psychologists drive expensive cars. About 10 to 20 percent of erection problems are caused, at least in part, by psychological issues. Therapists who specialize in sexual problems such as impotence have a very high success rate at restoring normal performance.

EXERCISE DAILY. No kidding, it makes a difference. For one thing, regular exercise, even if it's nothing more strenuous than walking for half an hour, improves bloodflow throughout the body, including in the penis. It also stimulates a surge in endorphins, those "happy" brain chemicals that dispel stress and make you feel mentally strong and confident—the keys to good sex.

THE ORGASMIC EDGE

An orgasm is one of those ineffable sensations that are impossible to put into words. So we won't even try; you know what it feels like. The issue for most men is how to control the timing of orgasms a little better, giving yourself and your partner a little more pleasure.

If you find that you come more quickly than you want to—keeping in mind that uncommonly steamy sex can give any man a hair trigger—you can literally train your penis to respond a little more slowly. In other words, it takes practice.

It's true. Men who deliberately take themselves through the whole sexual cycle—arousal and erection followed by a controlled orgasm—can learn to hold off to a surprising degree. You don't want to take this too far, of course. Myths to the contrary, most women don't appreciate a man who tirelessly pounds away like a piston. It makes them sore, not excited. But ejaculatory control—whether that means lasting 5 minutes or 30—is one of the best gifts you can give yourself and your lover.

You can certainly improve ejaculatory control with lovemaking, but practice during masturbation is more effective because you can concentrate entirely on your body's responses rather than being distracted by the needs of your partner. The idea is to make masturbation a long, disciplined process, one that deliberately slows the sprint to orgasm. Here's what to do.

GIVE YOURSELF TIME. A lot of time. If you're like most men, you probably masturbate quickly, more to get rid of sexual tension than to languorously enjoy every moment. This approach almost guarantees a quick release—and trains your body accordingly.

TURN THE PROCESS AROUND. The next time you're in the mood, allow at least as much time for masturbation as you would if you were having sex with your partner. Foreplay with yourself? Why not? Set the mood: Dim the lights; spin some tunes. Touch yourself lightly, even casually at first. Savor the first tinglings of excitement. Once you're hard, see how long you can stay that way without coming. Keep the hot mental images flowing through your head, but don't let them take you over the top.

SQUEEZE TO STOP. When you feel that you're reaching the point of no return, stop doing whatever it is you're doing and firmly squeeze the frenulum, the sensitive part of the penis just below the head. Maintain the pressure until you no longer feel that you're about to come. Then s-l-o-w-l-y resume the strokes that got you there in the first place.

TAKE YOURSELF FORWARD AND BACK. Keep touching yourself until you feel like you're almost ready to come, then back off by squeezing the frenulum. Repeat the process at least two or three times—more often as you gain more control. The idea isn't only to delay your orgasm at the moment but also to train your body's responses to sexual stimulation. Just as you can lift progressively heavier weights every week that you go to the gym, you can train the penis to respond more slowly and with better control.

TAKE THE LESSONS TO REAL LIFE. The next time you're having sex, whether that involves touch, oral contact, or intercourse, practice the same start/stop technique. When you're about to come, grip the top of your penis, squeeze until the anticipatory feelings of orgasm fade, then start again.

You'll probably need to use the squeeze technique for awhile. Eventually you'll also gain more *mental* control of impending orgasms. Your penis—and the brain signals that fire it—won't demand the same immediate release that they did before. You'll last longer just by wanting to. That's good news for you and your partner.

When things don't work out as planned, as inevitably happens, put it out of your head. Too many men get so wound up by worries about sexual performance that they simply can't perform. Take seriously this advice from a 29-year-old woman, a newspaper reporter in Miami: *"Not being able to perform has a lot more to do with what's going on in your head than in your groin. If it's not happening, don't force it, and don't get upset about it. Tell me a fantasy that will get you going, and I'll act it out. Or just relax and let me*

SPANK YOUR CANCER RISK

Here's another argument in favor of masturbation: New research suggests that it may prevent cancer.

Australian researchers asked more than 2,500 men, ages 20 to 50, about their sexual habits. They found that those who ejaculated the most, more than five times a week, were a third less likely to get prostate cancer later in life.

Researchers speculate that ejaculation is a kind of flushing mechanism. A man's semen absorbs high concentrations of potassium, zinc, citric acid, and other substances from the blood. At the same time, it picks up potential carcinogens. A man who ejaculates frequently may be less vulnerable to cancer-causing cell changes.

The key seems to be masturbating; intercourse may not have the same effect. Ejaculation during sex with a partner does purge the prostate, but if you have multiple partners, you increase your risk of exposure to sexually transmitted diseases, which can increase prostate cancer risk by up to 40 percent.

give you a massage. The key is relaxing and getting your mind off it. Take away the pressure and let things happen naturally."

A TOTAL-CONTROL WORKOUT

One simple type of exercise, traditionally recommended by doctors to women patients, can make a tremendous difference for men who ejaculate more quickly than they'd like. The exercises, known as Kegels, improve ejaculatory control and can make an erection stronger and harder.

LIMITED INSURANCE

A condom will greatly minimize the odds that you'll catch a nasty disease—but it won't reduce the risk to zero.

Even though condom manufacturers follow stringent quality-control guidelines, you're still talking about a micro-thin sheath of rubber. Snagging a condom with a sharp fingernail can breach the delicate barrier. So can putting on a condom too roughly. Rubber breaks down over time, so condoms that were perfectly good when you bought them might be less than reliable a few years later.

Even if you use a condom with all its integrity intact, there's always the chance that it will work its way off during sex. There is also the unpleasant possibility of an unforeseen explosion—not to mention infection from diseases that don't depend strictly on genital-to-genital contact, such as herpes or venereal warts.

To play it safe, you're better off using latex condoms than "skins." Synthetic materials have smaller pores, which reduce the risk that an elusive microbe will slip through. Pay attention to what you're doing when putting on a condom. Work gently, and definitely remove it as soon as you're done having sex. A condom that fits firmly on an erection is like a loose pair of jeans once you get soft.

First developed by Los Angeles gynecologist Arnold Kegel, M.D., the exercise is designed to strengthen the pubococcygeus (PC) muscle in the pelvis. The PC wraps around the base of the penis and the anus and reflexively contracts during orgasm. Making the muscle stronger makes it easier to delay orgasms and makes them stronger and more intense.

The exercise itself couldn't be simpler. All you have to do is contract the PC muscle—the same one that you'd use to stop the flow of urine in midstream. Hold the contraction for 2 or 3 seconds, inhaling as you squeeze. Relax for a moment, then squeeze again. Do the exercise in sets of 10 at first, then increase the number to 20 or 30 squeezes. Repeat the sequence several times a day.

Once you've developed strength in the PC, you'll find that it's easy to stop an orgasm just by contracting it. It's easier and more convenient than the "squeeze" technique for stopping an orgasm during masturbation. Another key difference is that Kegels not only delay orgasm but actually build muscle at the same time—an important point because about 85 percent of men can't have intercourse for longer than 3 minutes, largely due to an underdeveloped PC.

▼

"The good thing about masturbation is that you don't have to dress up for it."
—TRUMAN CAPOTE,
American writer

▲

To start a Kegels plan, here's what doctors advise.

GET INTO TRAINING. When you first start doing Kegels, you'll probably find that you're able to delay orgasm by only a slight margin, if that. That's okay. Like any workout, Kegels require persistent practice. If nothing else, you get in the habit of locating and contracting the muscles at the key time. Most men need to practice Kegels for at least 3 to 4 weeks before they notice significant changes in their ability to hold back.

DO THEM ALL DAY. Don't wait until you're having sex to start building the PC muscle. To build maximum strength, you need to do sets of Kegels at least three times a day, working up to about 300 forceful squeezes daily. Doing this for a month or two will greatly strengthen the PC. At this point, you'll notice improvements in your staying power as well as in the pleasurable force of your orgasms.

DO THEM ANYWHERE. You don't have to change into workout clothes to do Kegel exercises. You can do them anywhere: while sitting on the sofa watching TV, standing in a checkout line, or leaning over the sink and scrubbing 3-day-old pasta sauce out of your favorite pot.

SHAKE THINGS UP. Bored with simple Kegels? Push yourself a little harder with these variations:

▶ Slow Kegels. Tighten the PC and hold for a slow count of three. Relax, then repeat 10 or more times.

▶ Quick Kegels. Tighten and relax the PC as many times as you can in 10 seconds.

▶ Big-move Kegels. Tighten your entire abdomen and the pelvic floor muscle, then force the pressure outward by bearing down.

▶ Fluttering Kegels. Quickly tighten and relax the PC using a fluttering movement for 10 seconds. Relax for 10 seconds, then repeat.

TAKE THE TOWEL TEST. A pleasurable way to test the strength of the PC is to see how successful you are at pulling back from the brink of orgasm. Here's another self-test: The next time you have an erection, hang a small bath towel on your penis and try to move it up and down. You won't have any trouble if the PC is strong. You can also use this exercise to make the muscle even stronger. Can you raise and lower the towel 100 times? The same movement inside your partner will give her an added bit of pleasure.

ALLOW SOME DOWNTIME. Working the PC with Kegels, like any other form of exercise, can leave you a little sore at first. Some discomfort is normal, but why live with it? Do Kegels for a few days, then take a day off to allow the muscle to flush out accumulations of pain-causing lactic acid. Then start the program again.

POWER TO THE PELVIS

You can't build a house with a hammer alone, and you can't have great sex just because you have a strong erection. You also have to have strong supporting muscles, especially those that attach to the pelvic girdle, the bony arch that supports your legs.

Sex, as Elvis showed shocked parents a generation ago, is all in the pelvis. Your partner will notice the difference when you're strong and limber enough to swivel and twist. A strong pelvis means that you can hold sexual positions, especially those that involve sitting, for a longer time, without straining your back or depending on your arms for support.

As with any stretching program, you can do the following pelvic workouts pretty much anywhere, even on your office floor if you can get away with it. Better yet, do them with your partner. Women benefit from a stronger pelvis just as much as men do, and doing the stretches together will add an erotically charged dimension to your relationship.

STRETCHES: POWER TO THE PELVIS

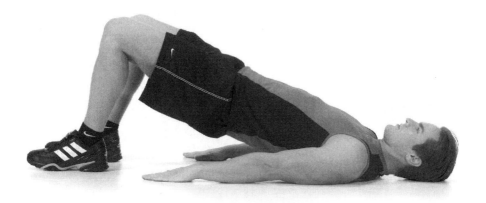

PELVIC LIFT

START: Lie on your back with your knees bent and slightly apart. Your feet should be flat on the floor and your arms at your sides.

FINISH: Inhale, firmly clench your abs and butt, and lift your pelvis until your spine is straight but not arched. Breathe out, hold for at least 10 seconds, then relax and repeat.

STRETCHES: POWER TO THE PELVIS

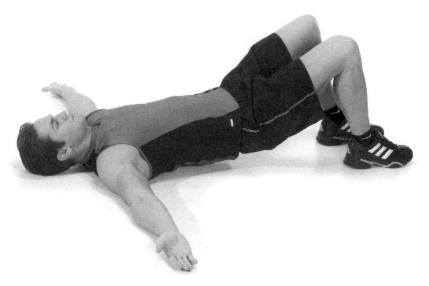

PELVIC BOUNCE

START: Lie on your back with your knees bent and slightly apart.
Extend your arms to the sides with the palms facing up.

FINISH: Inhale, lifting your pelvis just slightly off the floor. Hold for
a few seconds, then lower yourself so that your lower back lightly
touches the floor. Relax, then repeat. Exhale and let down so your
lower back bounces gently against the floor.

STRETCHES: POWER TO THE PELVIS

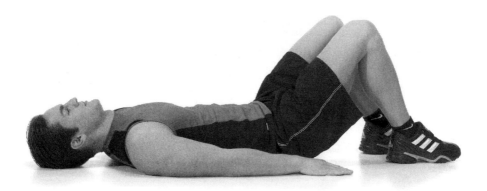

PELVIC TILT

START: Lie on your back with your knees bent. Your feet should be flat on the floor and your arms at your sides.

FINISH: Clench your abs and butt tightly while firmly pressing your lower back against the floor. Hold for 3 to 5 seconds, then relax and repeat.

STRETCHES: POWER TO THE PELVIS

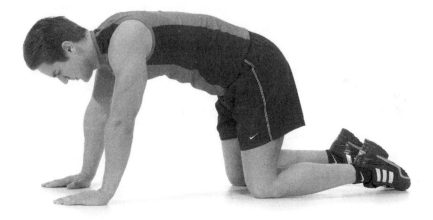

HORSE STANCE

START: Get on your hands and knees, with your elbows locked and your hands under your shoulder blades. Flatten your lower back and drop your shoulder blades.

FINISH: Pull your navel toward your spine and hold for about 90 seconds, then relax.

FINDING THE MULTIPLE O

Many women enjoy the unique pleasure of having multiple orgasms. This experience, alas, is denied to most men. When a man ejaculates, he naturally slips into a refractory period—the resting stage in which the body slowly prepares for more action. He's down for the count, in other words.

But some men do have multiple orgasms. The secret to their enjoyment lies in the fact that orgasm and ejaculation are two distinct events. Within limits, many men can teach themselves to experience orgasms without the out-rush of semen. Retaining semen during orgasm is the secret to coming again—and with luck, again and again. Some men report having three or four orgasms in succession, without interruption or loss of sexual arousal.

Sex researcher Dr. Alfred Kinsey estimated that the average man thinks about sex roughly every 5 minutes.

The ability to come repeatedly isn't as elusive as you might think. Then again, not every man can do it. It's really determined by the roll of your individual physiological dice. But anything that feels so good is certainly worth a try. Here's what you need to do.

GET COMFORTABLE. *Real* comfortable. A study by Marian E. Dunn, Ph.D., of the State University of New York Health Science Center in Brooklyn, found that most multi-orgasmic men had sex with women they knew well and were comfortable with. They also had their best moments when the atmosphere and circumstances surrounding sex were relaxed and stress-free. At the same time, it's helpful to periodically stimulate the entire penis, along with the scrotum and the perineum (the area between the anus and penis), to heighten sexual arousal.

STRENGTHEN THE PCS. They have to be strong to hold back the rush of semen when you come. Doing frequent Kegels throughout the day is essential if you hope to ride the multi-train.

SQUEEZE LIKE HELL WHEN THE MOMENT COMES. Either clench the PC when you feel an orgasm is imminent or use your hand to squeeze the top of your penis. You have to stop yourself from ejaculating, however tempting it might be to let go.

FOCUS ON THE SENSATIONS. Once you're able to back off when you're ready to come, pay special attention to what you're feeling. You may notice what experts call contractile phase orgasms, sensations that are very similar to, if more subtle than, regular orgasms. With practice, these "mini-orgasms" may be just as powerful as your former orgasms, with the special bonus of lasting longer.

CHAPTER 6

MASTERING TOTAL CONTROL

WE RECENTLY HEARD FROM A 47-YEAR-OLD FIREFIGHTER IN OMAHA. He might be bragging a bit, but his note illustrates better than we ever could the connection between physical fitness and great sex: *"For the average couple, unless they're in great shape, I would think they would have a hard time achieving the duration, intensity, and number and type of positions that my girlfriend and I experience."*

There's no deep mystery about why spending a few hours a week in the gym enhances libido as well as performance. Working out lowers levels of stress hormones. It can transform your heart into a pounding drum and your arteries into forceful conduits. It increases energy, improves sleep, and boosts levels of testosterone. You've heard all of this before, but it's definitely worth repeating because we can all use a little convincing to get off the couch and do—*anything*.

Strength training and cardiovascular conditioning are just one part of fitness. You also need a high degree of *sexual* fitness if you hope to have the kinds of intimate encounters that can fill your head with fantasies. This is the one area where nearly all men need some help. Even if you're physically capable of having the kind of sex you want—you get easy erections, don't tire easily, and so on—you might not have the specific skill sets to make sex last as long as you'd like or have the kind of mind-blowing orgasms that you dream about.

In the following pages, we'll explain, step by step, how to dramatically increase sexual endurance. How to come exactly when you want and not before. How to increase orgasmic intensity so that it rivals the multiple orgasms some women take for granted. These aren't pie-in-the-sky fantasies. Scientists who study sex have developed very

BITS AND PIECES

No matter how many times you've been around the block, there's always something new, or at least unfamiliar, in the world of sex. We asked some of the country's top researchers to share some of the little-known sexual facts that they felt every man should know. Here are their top picks.

▶ Only about a third of women come during straight intercourse. So quit feeling guilty—and put your fingers, mouth, or vibrator to work.

▶ Few women appreciate overly long sexual sessions. Making love for more than 30 minutes often causes more soreness than excitement.

▶ The average man loses and regains his erection up to four times during intercourse.

▶ The average woman is stimulated by the periodic softening of a man's penis in her vagina.

▶ Most women want a man to stay inside them as long as possible after intercourse.

▶ Men (and women) almost *have* to fall asleep after sex because the adrenal glands release a burst of epinephrine after orgasm. Epinephrine causes a temporary increase in pulse, blood pressure, and blood circulation to the muscles, which is followed by profound relaxation.

specific techniques for breathing, ejaculatory response, and muscular control. Some of these exercises are derived from clinical studies of men's sexual responses. Others are refinements of ancient sexual practices. Used together, they can take you to places you probably can't imagine now—places to which, when you look back 10 years from now, will make you wonder how you managed to be satisfied before.

ORGASM ON DEMAND

Have you ever wondered what makes you hard? Not what actually triggers the process—that could be anything from the sight of a tight miniskirt to the sensations of jeans against skin—but how your body translates the initial "I want some of that" fantasies into mechanical action? Although it varies from one person to another, these are the four phases of male sexual response.

▶ 1. Excitement: When you first get turned on, electrical signals travel from the brain down the spinal cord and into your genitals. Blood vessels relax, and blood pours into the spongy tissue in the penis. (Two chambers of tissue, the corpora cavernosa, wrap around the top and sides of your penis; a third chamber, the corpus spongiosum, wraps around the urethra and forms the head at the top of the penis.)

▶ 2. Plateau: Once enough blood is assembled—and for men over about age 40, this generally requires direct physical stimulation in addition to erotic thoughts—nerves in the genitals release a substance that essentially shuts the gates. Rather than flowing in and out as usual, blood stays in the spongy caverns. That's what makes you hard and keeps you hard until you ejaculate.

When you're approaching the point of no return, the prostate gland, the small band that circles the urethra at the base of the bladder, tightens, then releases fluid into the urethra. At the same time, the scrotum tightens, and the testicles jam up against the body. This is the moment when you're ready to go; it's like the split second after your finger pulls the trigger on a gun and sends a bullet toward the light of day. Nothing short of instantaneous death (and maybe not even that) will stop you from coming.

▶ 3. Orgasm: The pelvic muscles tighten and force semen out of the penis. All of that accumulated blood starts to ebb. Your heart pounds, and your breathing gets heavier and faster. Blood rushes to the skin and makes you feel hot and sweaty. All the while, you're out of your head with bliss because the orgasm, for those few precious seconds, has transported you to another realm.

▶ 4. Resolution: The body returns to its prearoused state. Men generally experience a "refractory period" at the beginning of resolution, during which achieving another erection is all but impossible.

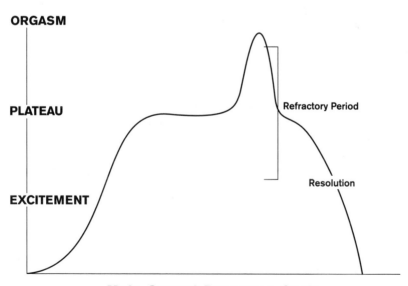

Male Sexual Response Cycle

The mechanics of orgasm are pretty straightforward, but the ability to control it is not. On the male anxiety meter, the idea of coming too quickly can blast you into the red zone, just behind the idea of not getting an erection. It's not a misplaced fear. Premature ejacula-

5 ANCIENT PLEASURE SECRETS

By taking the pressure off performance and enhancing sexual intimacy, ancient Tantric sex rituals have a great deal to offer couples today. These five are based on the 2,000-year-old body of erotic wisdom.

Ritual. Create a personal ritual to both celebrate and give special meaning to the sexual exchange. This might include candles, colored lights, flowers, perfumes, or a special room or bed. Also, consider expressions of affection like sensual massage or reciting poetry, or even reading erotica to each other.

Synchronized breathing. While touching your partner in some way, bring your breathing into sync with hers in order to create a feeling of relaxation and togetherness. Don't try too hard; instead use a "soft-focus" approach whereby you simply allow your breathing patterns to come together naturally.

Sustained eye contact. Though it may feel awkward at first, sustained, steady eye contact has tremendous potential for enhancing your sexual experience. Start out by doing it for a minute or two at a time, then continue as you get more comfortable with it.

Motionless intercourse. After you've entered her and are at a point of peak sexual arousal, become completely still. Start by doing this for a couple of minutes, then continue for longer periods.

Refrain from orgasm. To take the focus off performance completely, try lovemaking without orgasm. Tantric tradition suggests that avoiding or refraining from sexual release intensifies sexual/spiritual energy.

tion is among the most common problems sex therapists treat. Some men come almost immediately after entering their partners, and this can cause real problems—not only for a man's self-confidence but for his relationships as well. (See chapter 13 for more on ejaculation difficulties.)

Most men, though, last long enough for satisfying sex. Do they last long enough for great sex? Not often enough. The ability to *decide* when to come gives you a tremendous amount of freedom. There will be times when you and your partner, overcome by the heat of the moment, want nothing more than to explode into oblivion, the quicker the better. There will be many other times when you want to prolong the sensations, to explore a variety of positions, and to keep going and going.

Not a problem. The ability to last has very little to do with willpower and almost everything to do with technique and habit. Forget for the moment that longer sex may be its own reward. Men who train themselves to linger on the path to orgasm, who push themselves to the brink and then pull back repeatedly, generally experience greatly intensified pleasure. From a woman's point of view, your ability to last is a great bonus because it can allow her to come first while still feeling your erection inside her.

THE TANTRIC EDGE

Unless you've taken the time to really read up on the subject, most of what you've heard about Tantric sex probably should be filed under misinformation. In essence, it's a philosophy, science, and art that promotes the creative use of sexual energy. In India, the practice of Tantric sex was first codified in the love manual *Kama Sutra* and later developed into a series of ritualized sexual positions (tantras).

In a nutshell, Tantric philosophy teaches that lovemaking, when entered into with full awareness, opens a gateway to both sexual and spiritual bliss. It treats sexual energy as something to be prolonged and savored, rather than as a performance and race to orgasm. As you might expect, the ability to control ejaculation plays a key role in Tantric sex. Men who practice it say they routinely experience multiple orgasms. Orgasm can easily be delayed half an hour or more. In the Tantric view, this languorous approach to lovemaking not only enhances pleasure but also channels sexual energy into other pursuits in life, giving more energy and self-awareness.

▼

Until the U.S. Supreme Court struck down the nation's sodomy laws in 2003, the United States had more statutes governing sexual behavior than all the European nations combined.

▲

You could easily spend months learning the intricacies of Tantric sex. For our purposes, the bottom line is that you can incorporate some of the approaches into your daily life to enhance all of your sexual experiences. Here are the most important steps.

EXPAND YOUR EROTIC SENSES. Forget the bedroom for a moment. You can't be fully sensual in bed unless you also appreciate all of life's sensuous pleasures: the silky texture of a rich, creamy soup; the brush of the wind across your face; the striking colors of autumn leaves. A man who's in touch with all of his senses, and who takes time to savor them, is a man who also knows how to appreciate the sensations of his body and those of his partner. Sex doesn't begin and end with the penis. At its best, it's an all-day affair, a kind of ongoing mental foreplay that keeps you buzzing.

MASTURBATE OFTEN—AND TAKE YOUR TIME. Forget the businesslike speed and force you're probably accustomed to. Men tend to masturbate to "take the edge off," which basically means going hard at it until they come. This approach certainly works if your goal is to have an orgasm in the shortest possible time, but it leaves a lot to be desired if you hope to expand your self-awareness and potential for pleasure.

The next time you masturbate, slow w-a-y down. Light a few candles. Oil up your arms and chest, enjoying the slick sensations as you rub and massage. When you move your hands to your penis, go slowly. This isn't a race. Pay attention to your emotional as well as physical feelings. More important, notice how good you feel even when you're not even close to coming. Forget the destination. Forget old habits. Good sex means throwing predictability out the window. Subtle sensations are often the most powerful, especially when you give yourself time to really explore them.

BREATHE FOR ENDURANCE. Most of us breathe the same way we eat: automatically, without much thought. But in Tantric sex, conscious breathing can become part of the sensual experience because it makes you intimately aware of your body. The next time you're making love, make an effort to breathe much more slowly and deeply than usual. Pay attention to each breath as it goes in and out. Apart from heightening your physical sensations, deep breathing is among the best ways to dispel the buildup of tension that can rush you too quickly to ejaculation.

MAKE SLOW LOVE. The best sex is meditative and very intimate. The goal isn't to maximize sensations in your penis and come quickly. Quite the opposite. You and your partner should be as relaxed as possible. Even if you're inside your partner, move as slowly as you know how. As your erotic energy builds, take a break for awhile. Give your partner a sensual massage and encourage her to caress you before starting intercourse again. Get used to savoring all of the experience, not just the climactic end.

CLIMB THE FOUR STEPS. The goal of Tantric sex is for lovemaking to last as long as possible by building up and backing off repeatedly. Tantric devotees refer to the "four levels of ascent": As you make love, feel your sexual energy rising, starting with your navel and traveling upward to your heart, throat, and head. When you feel that the energy is entering the highest parts of your brain, that's the time to really let go. Men who practice this technique sometimes experience a "white light" orgasm. They feel the full, explosive rush, but don't ejaculate. With practice, you can learn to have several of these orgasms before you finally ejaculate.

HOW MUCH VARIETY DO YOU REALLY NEED?

There are nearly as many sexual positions as there are creative couples who like to say, "Let's try this!" If you spend any time perusing the Web or erotic classics such as the *Kama Sutra,* you might get the impression that your sex life is, well, vanilla if you don't spend your Saturday nights swinging from the swag lamp.

For some people—usually the same ones who never order the same dish twice at their favorite restaurant—variety really is the spice of life. Many others, though, will regularly return to a favorite restaurant because they can get the same delicious meal they had before. They're certainly game to try something new, but for the most part, they stick to the tried and true.

So too with sex. The majority of couples stick with the same few positions that have served them well in the past and that they continue to enjoy. There's nothing boring about that.

For those adventurous souls who spend their lives seeking out the more arcane pleasures, who enjoy things most when they're obscure as well as difficult, a quick word of caution: Some of the couplings you see on porn sites are challenging, to say the least. Be careful about exploring the outer limits of sexual acrobatics unless you're also willing to devote the time to staying impressively toned and limber.

KNOW YOUR BODY

We've talked at some length about Tantric sex because too many of us get locked into our habitual sexual responses and forget that we have the power to make them whatever we want them to be. The sexual wisdom of the East is one approach for taking control, but it's just one of many. Scientists have studied male sexual techniques and training exercises for decades. We're not talking about fuzzy concepts that are useful only if you spend your days meditating. They're very practical steps men can take to delay ejaculation and generally enjoy sex more fully.

The main reason that so many men come before they're ready is that they've never taken the time to know their bodies—to recognize the signs that say, "Whoa, it's gonna be over if I keep going." We all know what it feels like to come, but what about 30 seconds before you come? Or 2 minutes? Or 10? Having an orgasm isn't like falling off a building, even if it feels that way. A lot goes on before you get there. Once you recognize the earliest signs that the end is near and learn a few techniques for pulling back, you'll discover endurance you never knew you had. Which means more time to revel in all of the emotional and physical feelings.

The clinical term *ejaculatory inevitability* describes the point at which you're going to come, no matter what. It's during the time just before this point that you still have room to negotiate. For example, you'll probably notice these signs.

▶ Increased heart and respiratory rates. Apart from the loud breathing and pounding heart that accompany orgasms, you'll notice very gradual increases in both as your arousal rises. Unless you start out in an over-the-top state of heat, your breathing and heart rate will be close to normal when you first start making love. As the sensations get more and more pleasurable, your cardiovascular system significantly picks up the pace. This is the time to start slowing down.

▶ Contraction of the urethra. This one's pretty subtle, but you won't have any trouble feeling it when you pay attention. As you approach ejaculatory inevitability, the urethra—the tube that carries semen out of the penis—will go into pleasurable spasms. Once this happens, you don't have a lot of time. Basically, you'll have to stop whatever you're doing *immediately* if you hope to prolong the act.

▶ Increased penis size. Yep, you get bigger and usually harder as you approach orgasm. Again, you don't have a lot of time to back off once this happens—probably not much more than a few seconds if you don't slow down.

Apart from noting the sensations that accompany the climb to orgasm, it's worth keeping track of what you were doing that got you there. You probably have a good idea of the positions or movements that take you over the brink. Obviously, hard and fast sex—deep penetration and a lot of friction—will get you there fastest. The man-on-top position, because it provides the most stimulation, can trigger an early bailout for most men. The only way to truly control and expand your endurance is to get a good handle on what sets you off—and switch gears when the time is right.

THE POWER OF BREATH

We've already touched on the concept of breathing as an important tool when you're trying to increase endurance. It's worth exploring in more detail because breathing properly—yes, there is a *right* way to do it—is among the best ways to slow your body's rush to the finish line.

Most of us use less than one-third of our lung capacity when we breathe. This means that your body, including the penis, spends most of its life on reduced oxygen rations. Since men tend to breathe quickly and shallowly during sex, especially when they get close to orgasm, the penis is starved of air right when it needs it most. This isn't a minor point. Your cells demand oxygen. Reduce the supply, and all of the cellular processes, including those that govern the expansion of arteries and permit the circulation that makes you hard, take a sudden dive in efficiency.

The mere fact that you breathe in and out doesn't count for much. You can vastly improve your air supply—and your ability to come when you want and not before—with a few quick steps.

BREATHE YOURSELF HARD. Before you have sex—or during, if your partner sits on top and straddles your penis—lie on your back and breathe slowly through your nose. At the same time, put your hand on your pelvis and feel it slowly rise and fall. This simple move increases arousal levels while bringing more blood to the penis.

TIME YOUR THRUSTS. If you spend any time at the gym, you already know that you gain power and improve oxygen intake when you exhale during the exertion phase and inhale when you relax. The same with sex. Get in the habit of thrusting inward when you exhale and breathing deeply when you pull back. You'll vastly increase your oxygen flow while at the same time gaining a significant jump in energy. As a bonus, this type of synchronized breathing dispels muscular tension and can help you hold off before coming.

VISUALIZE AIR. Studies have shown that you can use a technique called visualization—in which you form vivid mental images in your mind—to enhance the circulation of oxygen-rich blood to your penis as well as to muscles in your arms and legs. The same technique can also enhance the intensity of orgasms. Once a day, take about 10 minutes to do the following exercise.

▶ Lie on your back with your knees bent and your feet flat on the bed.

▶ Breathe slowly and deeply for a few seconds, then start to visualize the air entering your bloodstream and flowing into your penis. Imagine that you can feel an increase in vigor and strength.

That's all there is to it. Studies have consistently shown that athletes who practice mental imagery have better concentration as well as performance. Visualization has also been shown to significantly lower stress hormones and improve blood pressure—and good blood circulation, as you know, is essential for good sex. Not bad for a 10-minute "workout" that's all in your mind.

Incidentally, you don't have to wait until you're in bed or lying on the couch to practice deep breathing or visualization. You certainly shouldn't wait until you're already in bed with your partner. You can easily incorporate both practices into your daily life whenever you have a few seconds of downtime—while you're waiting for a light to change, in the interminable line at the bank, and so on.

COME SLOWER, COME MORE

We talked a bit about techniques for achieving better ejaculatory control in chapter 5. They're *not* just for men who suffer from premature ejaculation. Even if your endurance is good—if, say, you can easily last 15 minutes during intercourse—you can use the same strategies to prolong lovemaking even more.

The cornerstone of any program to delay ejaculation is to repeatedly push your body to the brink and then pull back, repeating the process as often as you're able (or want to). If you do this regularly, you'll notice a dramatic improvement in your ability to "hold," possibly in as little as a few weeks. You'll probably start having orgasms that are almost mind blowing in their intensity. More than a few men who try these techniques start having multiple orgasms as well.

Here are the best techniques for ejaculatory control. Don't stick to just one; combine them for better—and faster—results.

STEP 1: STOP AND SQUEEZE. This is the easiest technique to delay ejaculation, although it may feel a bit unnatural at first. When you're masturbating or having sex, and you feel yourself reaching the point of orgasm, immediately stop what you're doing and firmly squeeze your penis just below the head. Continue the pressure for 15 to 30 seconds or until the urge to come subsides. Take a few deep breaths, then start again with whatever you were doing before.

> ▼
>
> **The average male produces a teaspoonful of ejaculate when he comes. The protein-rich dollop contains only 5 to 25 calories.**
>
> ▲

Keep doing this—squeezing when necessary, breathing a few times, then resuming—until you're finally ready to come. Men who practice this technique regularly can often mentally pull themselves back from the brink without having to squeeze the penis each time. Of course, this works only if you stop and squeeze before you're slipping over the edge into orgasm.

STEP 2: STOP AND GO. When you're making love and feel that you're about ready to come, push your penis into your partner as far as you can, then stop—really stop. Press hard so that your pubic bone presses against hers. Hold this position until the urge to come passes. Resume thrusting until, once again, you reach your peak, then back off again.

STEP 3: TENSE AND TEASE. This is a slightly advanced technique for delaying orgasm because it requires quite a bit of muscular strength and control. Shortly before you feel yourself coming, tense the muscles hard at the base of your penis. They're the same muscles that you'd use to stop the flow of urine. Maintain the pressure until the urge passes.

This step is the hardest for men to master because they might not have well-developed pubococcygeus (PC) muscles, which stop urine as well as the flow of semen through the penis. You can bet that you'll fail the first couple of times you try it. You can accelerate your learning curve by doing Kegel exercises most days of the week. Kegels (you'll find a complete workout program starting on page 133) greatly strengthen the PC and are an essential tool in gaining better ejaculatory control.

They actually do more than that. Men who strengthen their PC muscles with Kegels and get in the habit of tensing and teasing sometimes find that they're able to experience multiple orgasms. Clamping down the PC just prior to or even during orgasms can minimize or stop ejaculation. You'll still experience the pleasurable sensations of orgasm, but without the usual rush of semen. When you take ejaculation out of the picture, you may find that you're able to experience two or even three of these "mini-orgasms" in rapid succession.

STEP 4: PULL OUT AND STOP. Another method for learning ejaculatory control is called the locking method, and it's based not on Tantric philosophy but on another Eastern tradition, Taoism. Here's how it works. When you feel that you're becoming too excited, simply withdraw your penis from your partner's vagina or pull back so that only the head of your penis remains inside her, then stay motionless for 10 to 30 seconds. You'll begin to lose your erection, but if you wait until the urge to ejaculate begins to subside before entering her again, you'll also begin to learn ejaculatory control. You can do this as often as you like, until you begin needing to withdraw less and less often.

Taoist masters also advised novices to practice "a thousand loving thrusts" in a variety of styles. For instance, thrust in a pattern of three slow and shallow, then one fast and deep. If you start getting too excited, just withdraw and wait for it to pass, then resume thrusting. Once you've mastered this, move on to five shallow and one deep, then nine shallow, one deep.

A final word about delaying orgasm and heightening your sense of control: Don't underestimate the power of communication. Definitely talk to your partner about what you hope to accomplish. Don't worry, she'll be all for it. And you'll need her help when you're trying to hold back a little longer. If she's doing something that's too stimulating, ask her to back off a bit. When you're ready to resume again, let her know. Working together, you'll find a comfortable sexual pattern that gives all the pleasure that you're accustomed to—and more, because you'll have the ability to enjoy it longer.

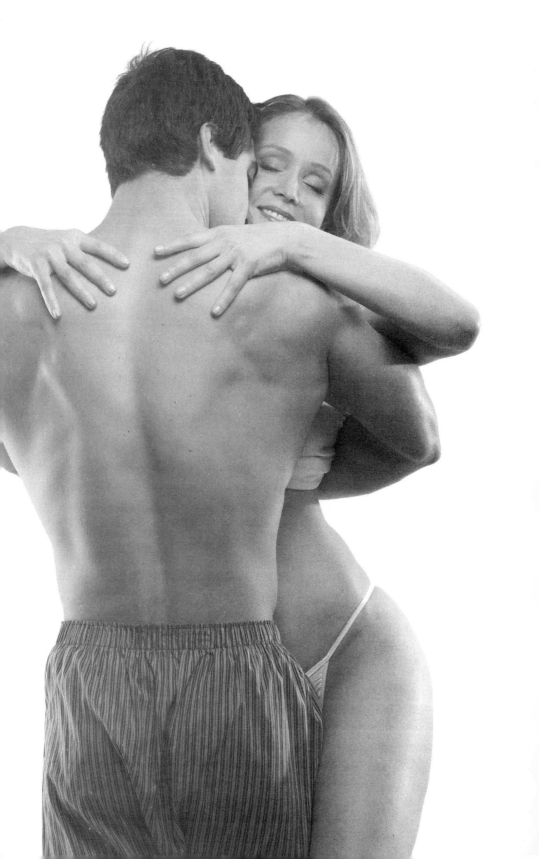

PART 3

SEXUAL FITNESS

CHAPTER 7

BEND THIS WAY:
THE ROLE OF FLEXIBILITY

**FLEXIBILITY IS ARGUABLY THE MOST IMPORTANT COM-
PONENT OF SEXUAL FITNESS, AND IT SEEMS TO BE THE
EASIEST ONE TO IGNORE.** Let's face it, there's a deep, gut-level
satisfaction in bench pressing your own weight and building a sexy
chest that women love, or running every weekend to strengthen
your thighs, or finding in yourself the determination to compete in
a 10-K race without clutching your chest and keeling over halfway
to the finish line. But stretching? B-o-r-i-n-g.

True, stretching lacks the drama and visceral thrill of competitive
exercise, which is why you don't see a lot of it on ESPN. Here's
something to think about, though. The benefits of flexibility go way
beyond strength and endurance. To put it simply, being limber
means more and better sex. You're more likely to play with new positions when your muscles move fluidly. You'll increase your
partner's pleasure as well as your own when you're comfortable
bending, twisting, tilting, and turning.

In less ecstatic terms, you're also less likely to get hurt when you're somewhat more limber than a saltine. Have you ever been tempted to manipulate your partner into the Hastika (elephant) pose from the *Kama Sutra* or simply to pull off a quickie in the front seat of a Neon? You'd better be flexible, or your only post-coital action will be in traction.

A letter from a *Men's Health* magazine reader amply (and painfully) illustrates this point: *"I've been trying to demonstrate to my significant other how much I appreciate her by going above and beyond in our lovemaking, but I've created a problem for myself. My desire outstrips my ability, and I end up with pains and cramps."*

Mmm, doesn't *that* sound like fun.

FLEXIBILITY GOES FIRST

If you're like most men, you've probably noticed that your body doesn't always respond the way you want it to or the way it used to. Forget about the obvious things for a moment, such as the sad fact that your erections aren't as hard as you remember or occur more slowly and less often. On the downhill slope, flexibility is right at the top—and it keeps sliding as the decades pass.

Exercise physiologists have long noted that flexibility peaks when you're somewhere between 10 and 15 years old. In fact, you start to lose flexibility a good 15 years before the usual age-related physical declines, such as drops in muscle mass and metabolism. If you're over 35, you've probably already found yourself saying things like, "Man, I'm stiff in the morning" or "Honey, would you help me pick up my socks?"

Don't make the mistake of confusing age-related stiffness with an inevitable law of nature. Flexibility, like any other physical skill, can always be improved. Put another way, a loss of flexibility is mainly a function of how you move—or, to be honest, how you *don't* move.

Stiffness doesn't just happen. It's a consequence of not regularly pushing your muscles through their full range of motion. When you don't flex regularly, in bed or anywhere else, your muscle fibers shorten, get tighter, and snap like angry dogs when you ask them to move.

"Simply being able to roll around while 'coupled' would be easier if we were both more flexible," says a 47-year-old firefighter. *"Some positions are difficult to maintain because of the awkward feelings that a lack of flexibility causes."*

It's normal, if not exactly smart, for men to focus on strength at the expense of flexibility. But you have to realize that the sexual advantages of strength, such as the ability to balance your partner on your thighs, are offset when movement is restricted by tight, stiff muscles. Sex relies much more on fluid motion than it does on brute strength. Stretching lubricates joints and makes tendons and ligaments more supple. In other words, it prepares you for the sensuous movements of sex.

▼

Eighty-five percent of all men ejaculate in 3 minutes or less.

▲

Here are other reasons to flex for sex.

▶ It takes only a few minutes a day, and you don't have to suit up to do it. You can even stretch with your partner before you get out of bed. Focus on shared, sensuous moments that take out the morning kinks—and that naturally transform themselves into foreplay.

▶ Stretching improves muscle growth and recovery from exercise (yes, even from sex), while at the same time enhancing sexual expression. Your muscles will work with you instead of against you.

▶ You'll feel increased sensitivity in all parts of your body when you're limber. And we do mean in *all* parts.

▶ A flexible man is a sexually creative man. You'll be more in tune with your body, more aware of what feels good—and what makes your partner feel good. Better still, you'll have the physical ability to act on your desires.

YES, SIZE MATTERS

Of course it does. Anyone who says that size doesn't matter is either lying or has been unduly influenced by the thought police. Let's face it, a man doesn't want to be so small that he gets, well, lost during sex. Nor does he want to be so large that he threatens injury.

Between these two extremes, it all comes down to a woman's preference. The average erect penis is 6.16 inches—perfectly adequate for the vast majority of women. There will always be exceptions, of course. Vaginas, like penises, come in different shapes and sizes, and they expand and contract to different degrees. Some women like a large penis because it offers a tighter fit. Others prefer a little more room to move.

Obviously, all is relative in this domain. A man who's too large for one woman will be perfectly sized for another. One who gets lost in one woman will be custom-fit for someone else. The bottom line: Average is about right. Besides, survey after survey reports that women are far more concerned with a man's technique and enthusiasm than with penis size.

One last point: Men often worry about the length of their penises, but it's the girth that makes a bigger difference. The lower third of a woman's vagina possesses the highest concentration of nerve endings. The wider the man, the more he'll fill this area.

Men determined to "go wide" can easily achieve this by wearing a penis ring, available in any adult "toy" store, during sex. It's like tying a string around your finger. It traps more blood inside the penis, causing it to expand. If you go this route, though, be sure to get one that's adjustable, and take it off as soon as you're done having sex. You don't want to restrict bloodflow indefinitely.

▶ You'll have more energy. Stretching increases circulation. Better bloodflow means better erections and higher arousal levels. It can also improve your ability to take in oxygen and blow out carbon dioxide. Better breathing, as you learned on page 152, can even be the key to overcoming too-quick ejaculation.

▶ Regular stretching keeps muscles in balance, so that bones and joints are properly aligned. It's especially good for the "sexual core" muscles in the pelvis, hips, and abdomen— muscles that don't get much of a workout in an average day but are essential for comfortable and erotically charged moments.

It should be obvious by now that the benefits of stretching are hardly limited to the health club and that they extend beyond how you feel at any given moment. "When people stretch together, they become aware of each other's physical dimensions," says Paul Frediani, a personal trainer and former Golden Gloves champion. "Flexibility results in more freedom of movement during sex."

And that's the bottom line. Stretching will help you take sex to another level. Think of your favorite position. Now, imagine doing it with more flexibility and strength, with calmer nerves, greater vitality, and enhanced erotic energy. That's a whole lot of benefit from something that can take less time than wrestling with a tough condom wrapper.

SEXUAL GAIN WITHOUT PAIN

Sex is about pleasure. Pleasure usually means an absence of pain. A simple equation—but judging from the comments we got when researching this book, a lot of us haven't quite figured it out.

Consider this note from a 45-year-old certified public accountant: *"I find that as I get older, some positions can become uncomfortable after a length of time, and a muscle cramp can be very distracting."*

Or this one from a 24-year-old IT support specialist: *"I pulled a leg muscle once trying an awkward position."* And this from an 18-year-old college student: *"I feel like I'm about to pull a groin muscle when I have sex."* Then there's this from a 42-year-old insurance rep: *"I threw my back out during sex."*

What's going on here? These guys are in the primes of their lives, for gawd's sake! If you're having this kind of pain during sex when you're 18 or 24 or 42, can you imagine what whoopee's going to be like when you're 50 or 60?

▼

Surveys reveal that 98 percent of men would gladly increase the size of their penises if they knew a safe way to do it.

▲

You're a lot more likely to avoid the sorts of aches and pains, and in some cases out-and-out injuries, that can take you out of service between the sheets just by maintaining a supple body. Studies show that most men don't stretch at all during the day. Without a little prep work prior to penetration, you can bet that their sexual horizons are a lot more limited than they need to be.

In fact, some sex books advise men to literally take a few minutes in the bedroom for some presex stretching. Imagine the look on your partner's face when you say, "Excuse me, Honey"—then drop down on the carpet for some kind of Richard Simmons routine. *She'd* be the one getting cramps—from laughing so hard.

Not that some gentle stretching before sex is such a bad idea. But what you really need to be doing, and what makes a lot more sense in real life, is to set aside stretch time throughout the day. Timing doesn't matter very much. Muscles have memory: The stretching that you do in the morning or on your lunch break will pay off hours later when the lights go down.

But you have to stretch smart. You might think of stretching as "exercise lite," but if you do it without a little warmup and preparation, you aren't going to get limber, and you emphatically won't have better sex. Why? Because you'll get hurt. Here's what you need to do instead.

RAISE YOUR BODY TEMPERATURE. Yes, you'll need to warm up before doing any stretch, even the easy ones. In fact, it's just as important to warm up before stretching as it is prior to hard-core running or lifting. A warmup does just that: It raises your body temperature. A cold human body, like unheated plastic, breaks down during movement if it isn't warmed to sufficient pliability.

So before you stretch, do some simple, light moves. Walk for a few minutes. Stride from room to room. Swing your arms or do high knee lifts. Rotate your legs, your hips, your arms. A few minutes is enough. A rule of thumb: If you *feel* warm, you're warm enough to start stretching.

FIGURE OUT WHAT YOU'RE DOING. *Duh,* you say. But you'd be amazed how many men don't know how to stretch. They wind up doing the same moves—usually the wrong ones—that they see other guys doing at the gym. Think about this for a moment. How many of those guys would you trust to give authoritative advice on cardiovascular surgery or accounting or legal ways to keep the couch during a messy divorce? The ability to bench 280 pounds doesn't confer knowledge. When you stretch wrong, you can actually tear muscle fiber. Torn muscles can leave behind tough scar tissue that can elevate pain and stiffness to levels you don't want to contemplate.

At the very least, take the time to read some fitness books (including this one) and look closely at the stretching illustrations and instructions. Better yet, set up a meeting with a trainer. Most gyms include a session or two as part of the cost of membership. The benefits of smart stretching aren't limited to injury prevention. You'll probably wind up saving time as well because you'll learn how to get the most efficiency from each move.

MAKE THE COMMITMENT. Sorry, stretching isn't like winning the lottery. You have to keep punching your ticket, or you'll wind up like the Tin Man without WD-40. The only way you'll stay flexible is to keep working at it. You brush your teeth every day. Stretching deserves the same commitment, especially when you consider the erotic payoffs.

DUMP THE TYPE A. This is the hardest message to get across. Muscle work, like it or not, takes time. You can plan on stretching for at least a week before you'll notice any real difference in how you move. After that, it will be at least a month, and probably more, before you achieve anything resembling maximum flexibility—and before you fully reach your erotic potential.

STRETCHING SMART

Stretching is typically divided into two types: static and ballistic. You can pretty much forget about the latter. It requires you to bob or bounce while performing some activity, like touching your toes. This type of stretching forcibly stretches a muscle, using your own momentum to hyperextend the muscle beyond its normal limit.

These days, ballistic stretching is pretty much frowned upon, except possibly for gymnasts and ballerinas. Unless you're already in great shape and are planning to have sex on a trapeze, there's never a good reason to jerk a muscle beyond its usual range of motion. It won't improve your performance in bed, and you'll probably spend the rest of the week walking around like Groucho Marx.

Static stretches are a lot more useful and are less likely to send you to a chiropractor. In static stretches, the muscle is stretched only to the point where you start to feel a pull. The idea is to extend the muscle almost, but not quite, to the point of discomfort. Going farther than that will tear tiny muscle fibers, damaging the area that you're trying to loosen and strengthen.

A simple example of a static stretch is to sit on the floor with your legs extended and reach forward to grab your toes. No bouncing or jolting—just a slow, steady pull.

Regardless of the specific stretches that you actually do—we've included static stretching programs for beginning, intermediate, and advanced levels—you want to hold each one for about 30 seconds. Trainers used to advise men to hold stretches for only 5 to 15 seconds, but studies have since shown that isn't anywhere near long enough to extend the muscle. In fact, it's probably no better for flexibility than not stretching at all. So follow the 30-second rule. You'll actually save time because a stretch held for that long is about as efficient as it gets. Conversely, don't bother holding the stretch for longer. You might think you're getting extra benefit when you hold a stretch for a minute or more, but it doesn't seem to be any more effective than a 30-second stretch.

Stretching is fundamentally pretty easy stuff. You can do it in the privacy of your home. You don't have to pop for equipment, and you can do it just about anywhere. About the only caveat is to maintain good posture: neck relaxed; head held naturally and aligned with the spine; shoulders down and back; stomach in; and knees slightly bent, not locked.

But you do want to stretch consistently—at least two or three times a week. Start slowly, of course; don't bounce (save that for the bedroom); and breathe deeply and easily throughout. Do each stretch at least half a dozen times, and don't forget to hold it for the full 30 seconds. Stretching won't make you a sexual athlete overnight. What it will do is give you the physical ability to go wherever your sexiest fantasies take you. How's that for motivation?

PHASE 1 ▶

THE STRETCHES INCLUDED HERE ARE INTENDED FOR THE GUY WHO ISN'T A HARD-CORE ATHLETE—who wants to gain flexibility and strength in bed while at the same time being better able to perform comfortably in just about any of the usual positions. Each of the stretches in this section will also increase power in the chest, arms, back, and legs. If you're spending time in the so-called missionary position, for example, these stretches will help ensure that you don't get crippled by cramps. At the same time, they'll strengthen and give flexibility to muscles in the lower back and abdomen—necessary for comfortable thrusting.

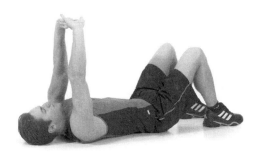

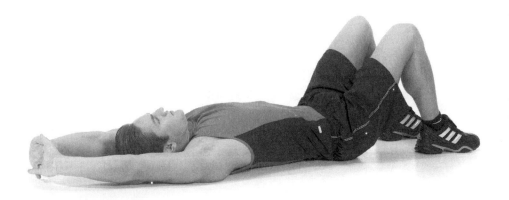

SHOULDERS

Lie on your back and extend your arms above your shoulders, perpendicular to the floor. Clasp your fingers together with your palms facing the ceiling. Keeping your arms straight, slowly lower them until your hands rest on the floor behind your head. Hold for 30 seconds, return to the starting position, and repeat.

▶*Sexual Gains:* **This stretch enhances your stamina in man-on-top positions by easing the toll on your shoulders.**

171

STRETCHES: PHASE 1

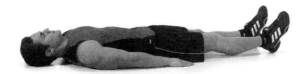

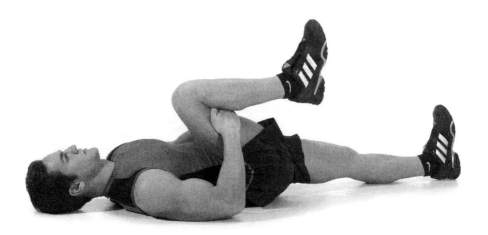

HIPS

Lie on your back with your legs straight. Grasp your right upper thigh with both hands and pull your right knee toward your chest. Hold for 30 seconds, return to the starting position, then repeat. Do the same thing with your left leg.

▶*Sexual Gains:* **Stretching the hips allows you to thrust stronger and longer.**

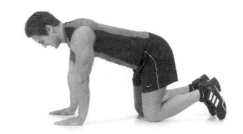

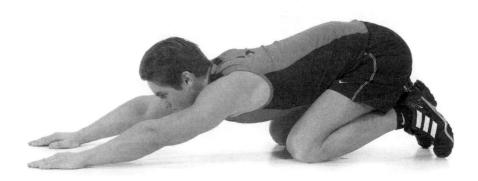

LOWER BACK

Get on your hands and knees, with your hands directly under your shoulders. Keeping your hands in place, sit back on your heels until you feel a stretch along your back; your arms will be outstretched at this point. Hold for 30 seconds, then repeat.

▶*Sexual Gains:* **Improves endurance and strength for kneeling positions and standing positions when you're supporting most of her weight and yours.**

STRETCHES: PHASE 1

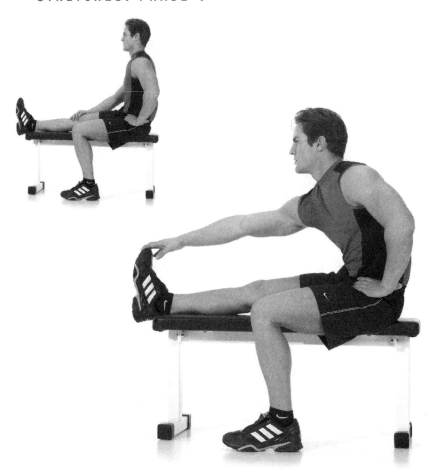

HAMSTRINGS

Sit on the edge of a bed or bench. With your left foot on the floor, raise your right leg and extend it. Put your right hand on your right knee and slowly slide it forward until you touch your toes—or as close as you can comfortably get. Hold for 30 seconds. Then stretch the left leg.

▶*Sexual Gains:* This exercise is better than similar stretches in which you sit on the floor because it puts less strain on the lower back. Flexible hamstrings improve your endurance and strength in standing and kneeling positions.

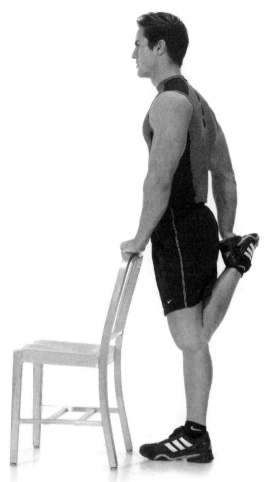

THIGHS

Stand, resting your left hand on a wall or the back of a chair for
support. Bend your left knee and grab your left foot with your right
hand. Pull your foot up until the heel presses against your butt.
Hold for 30 seconds. Repeat with the right leg.

▶*Sexual Gains:* **Flexibility in the front of the thigh
(quadriceps) will help you kneel for long periods and counter-
push when she's on top.**

STRETCHES: PHASE **1**

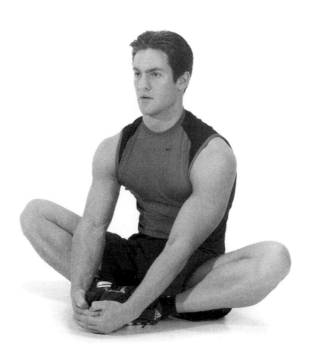

GROIN

Sit on the floor with your back straight. Draw your feet up to your body until the soles touch. Let your knees drop to either side, but don't overextend the muscles by letting them drop too far. Hold for 30 seconds, then repeat.

▶*Sexual Gains:* **Stretching the groin area allows for stronger thrusting and greater versatility in positioning.**

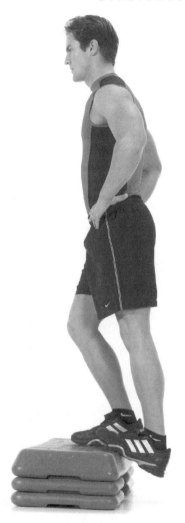

CALVES

Stand on a step and lower the heel of your left foot over the edge of the step until you feel a tug. Hold for 30 seconds. Repeat with your right foot.

▶*Sexual Gains:* **This stretch prevents the crippling cramps men sometimes experience from overflexing their calves during orgasm.**

STRETCHES

PHASE 2 ▶

LET'S ASSUME THAT YOU WORK OUT A LOT. MAYBE YOU RUN OR SWIM A FEW TIMES A WEEK OR LIFT WEIGHTS PRETTY REGULARLY. Or you've been doing the Phase 1 stretches for several weeks, and they are starting to seem easy and effortless. These stretches are a little bit harder than the ones in Phase 1, with a correspondingly greater payoff: You might find yourself attempting some sexual positions you haven't tried before—holding your partner and having sex while standing, to name just one tempting example.

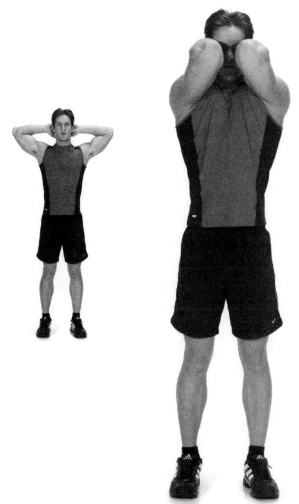

CHEST

Clasp your hands behind your head, with your elbows out to the sides. Inhale and exhale naturally while moving your elbows in front of your face. Hold the stretch, then move your elbows to the sides until you feel a stretch in your chest. Hold for 30 seconds, then repeat.

▶*Sexual Gains:* **Improves breathing capacity; helps you last longer when you're on top or during rear-entry sex when you're supporting yourself with your arms.**

STRETCHES: PHASE 2

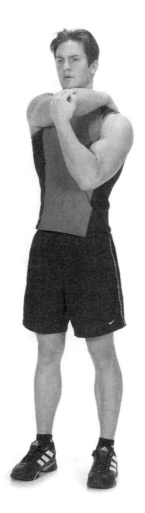

SHOULDERS

Grab the back of your right elbow with your left hand. Pull your right arm across your body and up and under your chin—or at least as far as you comfortably can. Hold for 30 seconds. Repeat with the left arm.

▶*Sexual Gains:* **Gives you better range of motion for reaching around and caressing your partner in positions where you're behind her.**

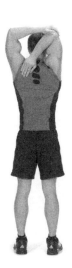
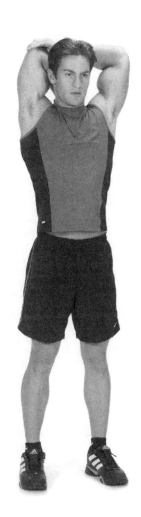

TRICEPS

Lift your right arm over your head and, with your left hand, gently push back on the right triceps, just above your elbow. Hold for 30 seconds, then repeat with the left arm.

▶*Sexual Gains:* **Improves arm stamina during man-on-top sex and while performing manual stimulation.**

STRETCHES: PHASE 2

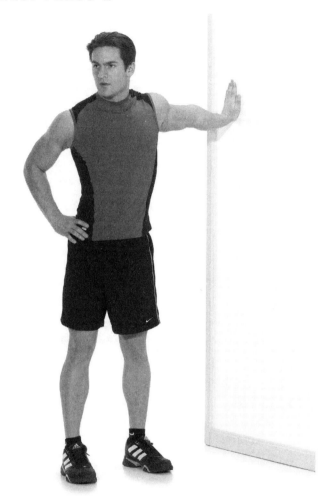

BICEPS

Rest your left hand against a wall. Turn your torso away from the wall and extend your arm as straight as you can, until you feel a stretch in the left biceps. Hold for 30 seconds. Repeat with the right arm.

▶*Sexual Gains:* **Improves endurance in standing and other positions when you're supporting her weight with your arms, and when performing manual stimulation.**

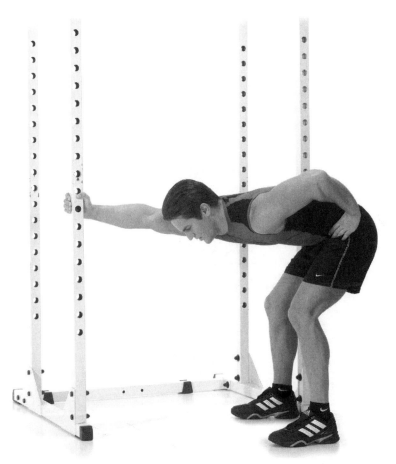

UPPER BACK

Find a sturdy bar (or a horizontal surface that's about chest high).
Stand about 3 feet away from it, bend at the waist, lean forward,
and grip the bar with your right hand. Lower your head and chest
until you feel a good stretch in your upper back. Hold for 30
seconds, then switch arms and repeat.

▶*Sexual Gains:* **Improves endurance and flexibility in
man-on-top positions and seated positions when you're leaning
forward, holding her up.**

STRETCHES: PHASE 2

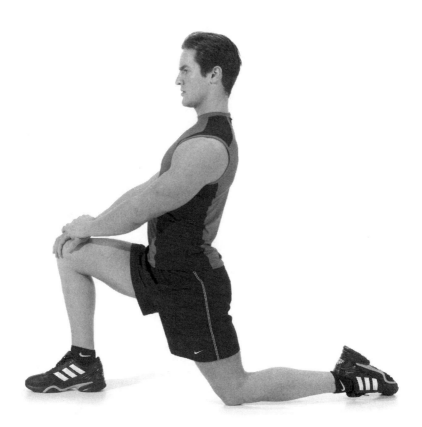

THIGHS

Kneel on your left knee with your right foot about 2 feet in front of you. Tilt your pelvis forward by tucking your glutes under your torso and pulling your belly button toward your spine. Place both hands on your right knee, then shift your body weight forward until you feel a stretch in the top of your left thigh. Hold for 30 seconds. Repeat with the left leg.

▶*Sexual Gains:* **Allows better range of motion in sitting and kneeling positions.**

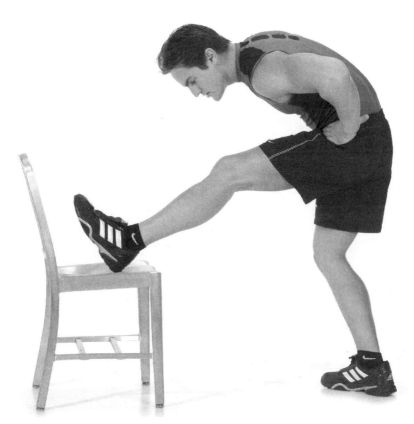

HAMSTRINGS

Rest your left foot on a chair and bend your torso over your leg as if you're trying to touch your knee with your forehead. Keep the knee slightly bent. Hold the stretch for 30 seconds. Repeat with the right leg.

▶*Sexual Gains:* **Gives you better range of motion for positions in which you're behind your partner or you're both standing and leaning over a table or bed.**

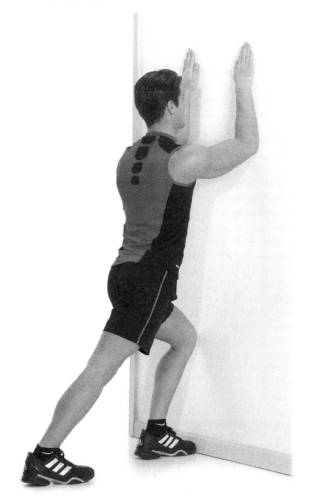

CALVES

Stand facing a wall and rest your forearms on it. Move your right foot back 3 to 4 feet. Bend your left leg, keeping your right leg straight. Keeping your right heel on the floor, lean even closer to the wall, until you feel a good stretch in your right calf. Hold for 30 seconds. Repeat with the left leg.

▶*Sexual Gains:* **Improves your range of motion and endurance for subtle tiptoe thrusts in man-on-top positions.**

STRETCHES

PHASE 3 ▶

YOU WON'T HAVE A WHOLE LOT OF TROUBLE WITH THE STRETCHES WE'VE DISCUSSED SO FAR. Now it's time for the next phase of the program, one that can push your muscles—and the sexual activity you'll use them for—into the stratosphere. Once again, each of these stretches focuses on the muscles you use most during sex. When you get through this program, you'll have flexibility you never dreamed of, along with more energy and a lot more sexual endurance.

Obviously, you don't want to attempt this program until you're already in good shape—at a minimum, after several weeks of doing the easier stretches.

STRETCHES: PHASE 3

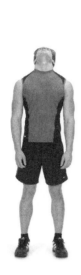
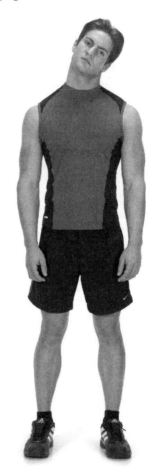

NECK

Relax your shoulders and drop your chin to your chest. Let it hang there for about 30 seconds. Raise your head slowly to an upright position and keep going, until you're looking at the ceiling. Hold it for 30 seconds, then return your head to level. Next, tilt your head so that your left ear moves toward your left shoulder. Keep your shoulders still. Hold the stretch for about 30 seconds, then slowly raise your head and repeat on the right side.

▶*Sexual Gains:* **Prevents neck and shoulder cramps and allows for greater range of motion when you're performing oral sex.**

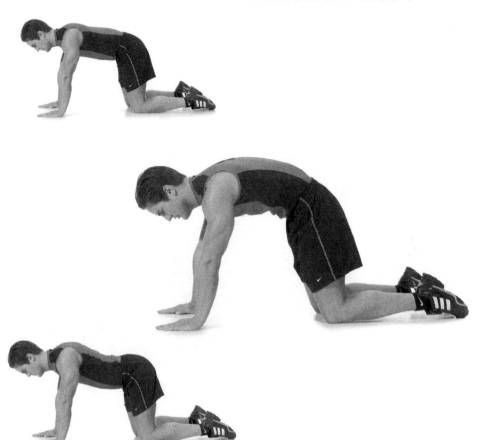

BACK

Get down on your hands and knees, with your back straight. Arch your back as high as you comfortably can. Hold for 30 seconds, then relax and repeat. Next, lower your belly, dropping your back as low as you comfortably can. Relax and repeat.

▶*Sexual Gains:* **Improves range of motion and endurance for mutual oral sex positions.**

STRETCHES: PHASE 3

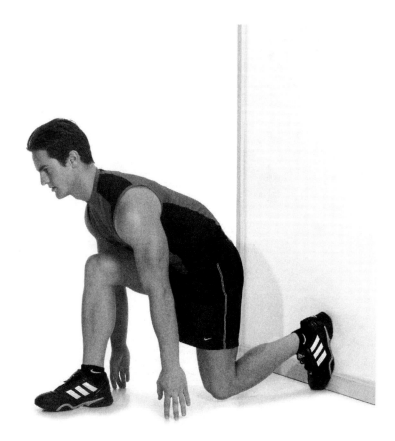

HIPS

Stand with your back about 2 feet from a wall. Extend your left leg behind you and press the heel against the wall. Bend your right knee and squat until your right thigh is parallel to the floor. Your right knee should be directly over your heel, so that your shin is at a 90-degree angle to the floor. Resting your fingertips lightly on the floor to keep yourself steady, press your left heel firmly into the wall, straightening your left leg while tightening the thigh muscles. Hold for 30 seconds. Repeat with the other foot.

▶*Sexual Gains:* **Improves hip-flexor range of motion so you can arch your back for maximum penetration.**

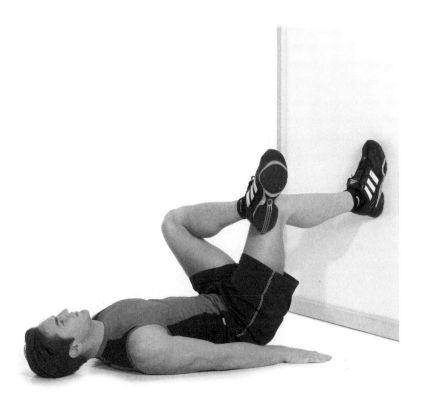

BUTT

Lie on your back, with your knees bent. Put your right foot on a wall, with the shin parallel to the floor. Place your left foot on your right thigh near the knee. (If the bottom of your spine lifts off the floor, move away from the wall until it rests firmly on the floor.) Hold the stretch for 30 seconds. Repeat with the other foot.

▶*Sexual Gains:* **Improves hip motion during thrusting.**

STRETCHES: PHASE 3

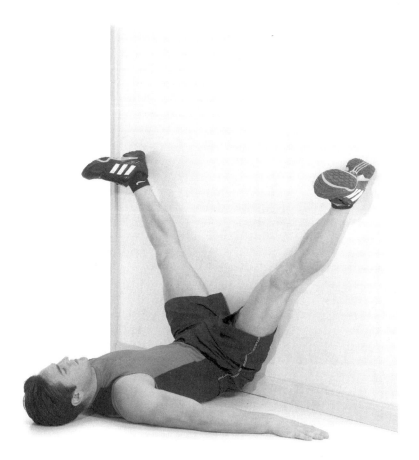

THIGHS

Lie on your back and extend your legs up a wall. With the back of your pelvis flat on the floor and your glutes resting against the wall, allow your legs to open slowly. Go as far as you comfortably can. Press the backs of your knees and legs against the wall. Let the full weight of your torso relax downward. If your knees hurt, bring your legs closer together. Hold the stretch for 30 seconds, then repeat.

▶*Sexual Gains:* **Increases stamina and range of motion in kneeling and standing positions.**

STRETCHING FOR TWO ▶

**THINK THAT EXERCISE ISN'T FUN? OH, HOW WRONG YOU
ARE**—when you exercise (maybe that should be "sexercise") with
your partner. There's certainly potential for fun, especially when
there's a good chance that the workout will wind up in bed.

The following stretching exercises are effective and reasonably
easy for just about everyone. We picked them specifically because
they lend themselves to increased flexibility in bed. At the same
time, they'll give you and your partner something to think about,
and who knows where that might lead?

Here's the thing: When you stretch with a partner, it's almost impossible not to talk about the experience. You need to tell each other
when a stretch is too much or too little; you'll also find yourself
talking about what you're feeling at the moment, physically as well
as emotionally. You don't need 17 sessions in couples' counseling to
know that the more you express your particular needs, the sexier
you're likely to feel. Talk during exercise naturally leads to talk
about sex, not to mention talk during sex. That can get pretty hot
indeed.

Of course, watching your partner move in exercise is enticing in
its own right. Mutual stretching allows you to be intimate with one
another without being sexual. Think of it as a kind of extended
foreplay.

The key to partner exercise is communication. Let each other
know how far to stretch and when to stop. As always, move slowly
and with total control, without bouncing or straining. Ease into
each stretch. Relax. Enjoy.

STRETCHES: STRETCHING FOR TWO

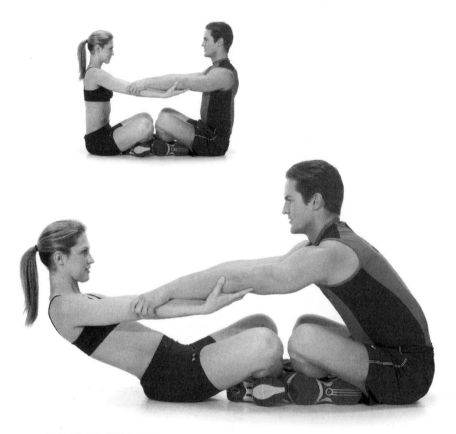

PULL IT TOGETHER

Sit on the floor facing your partner. Each of you should have your
legs crossed, with your knees nearly touching. Grip each other's
forearms in a way that is comfortable and allows you both to sit up
straight. Lean back slowly, gently bringing your partner toward you.
Be sure to keep your butt planted on the floor. Next, your partner
takes the lead, repeating the stretch. Hold each stretch for 30
seconds, then return to an upright position. Repeat five or six times.

▶ *Sexual Gains:* **Stretches the hips, lower back, and
shoulders, which improves endurance during seated sex, when
backs and shoulders tend to cramp and fatigue.**

STRETCHES: STRETCHING FOR TWO

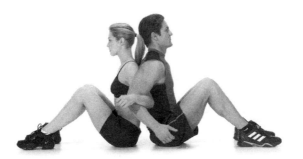

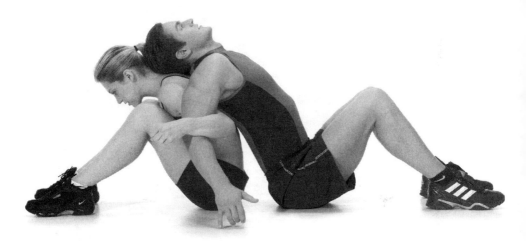

BACK TO BACK

Sit on the floor back to back. Your knees should be bent and relaxed, with your feet flat on the floor. Interlock your elbows with your partner's. Slowly lean forward, bringing your head toward your knees. Your partner should relax and allow herself to stretch back with you as far as is comfortable. Slowly return to an upright position. Next, your partner takes the lead, repeating the movements by leaning forward. Repeat five or six times, holding each stretch for 30 seconds.

▶ *Sexual Gains:* **Flexes the back muscles, allowing you to lean off the edge of the bed and say, "Ahh."**

STRETCHES: STRETCHING FOR TWO

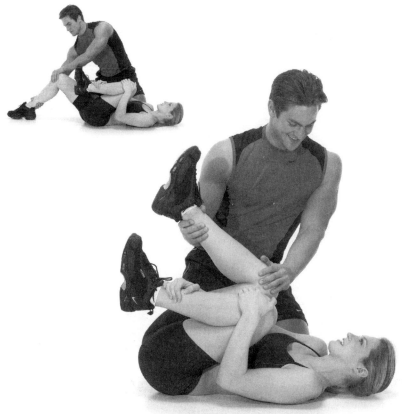

HIP FLEX

Lie on your back, with your right leg bent and your right foot flat on the floor. Your partner kneels on the floor at your right side. Grab your left knee and ankle with both hands. Your partner, meanwhile, holds your right knee and ankle, gently stretching the knee toward your chest while keeping the ankle in line with the knee. Exchange places with your partner. Hold this position for 30 seconds, then switch legs and repeat the stretch. Repeat two or three times.

▶*Sexual Gains:* **Maximizes your thrusting power and allows her to extend her legs all the way up and back for the deepest penetration.**

STRETCHES: STRETCHING FOR TWO

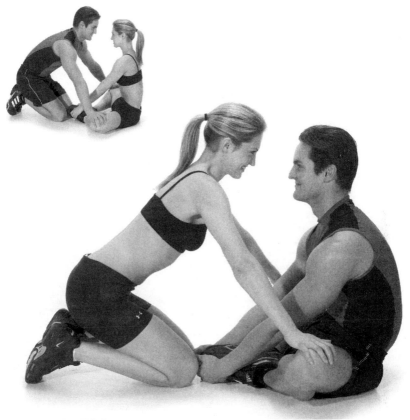

KNEE PRESS

Your partner should sit on the floor, with the soles of her feet together and her knees bent. Facing her, place your hands on her knees, and *gently* press them toward the floor. Then switch positions and let her take over. Hold each stretch for 30 seconds, then relax. Repeat five or six times.

▶*Sexual Gains:* **Stretches the inner thighs, improving comfort during sitting positions and range of motion for her to wrap her legs around you.**

STRETCHES: STRETCHING FOR TWO

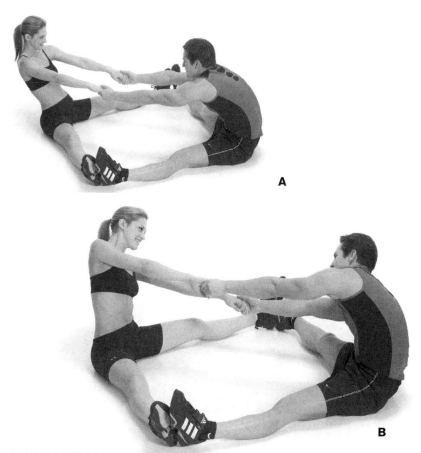

A

B

THE DIAMOND

Sit on the floor facing one another, with your legs extended in a comfortable V-shape. Press the bottoms of your feet against the bottoms of your partner's feet. Reach out and grip each other's hands. Next, while holding hands, have your partner slowly and gently lean forward, hold for a few seconds, then lean back. You, of course, follow.

Depending on your respective heights and your initial degree of flexibility, you may not be able to move more than an inch or two, but you will definitely feel the stretch in the back of your legs. After a bit, try leaning to the right, holding for a few seconds, then leaning

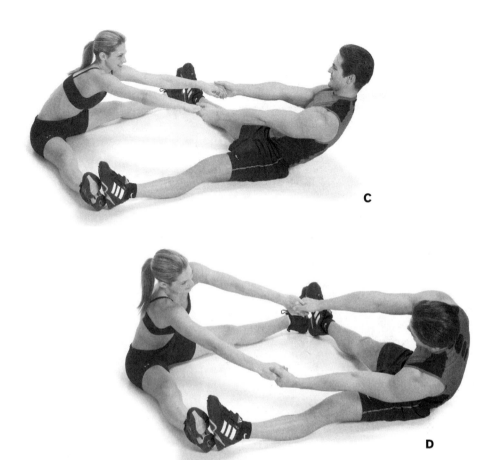

to the left. Next, try a circle: lean forward (A), to the right (B), back (C), and to the left (D). Keep going.

Take this one slowly and gently, until you've both achieved some flexibility. And don't push it: The stretch becomes counterproductive if you cause pain in the person with the shorter legs.

▶*Sexual Gains:* **Stretches the hamstrings, inner thighs, and calves, providing better endurance and range of motion in standing, kneeling, and sitting positions.**

STRETCHES: STRETCHING FOR TWO

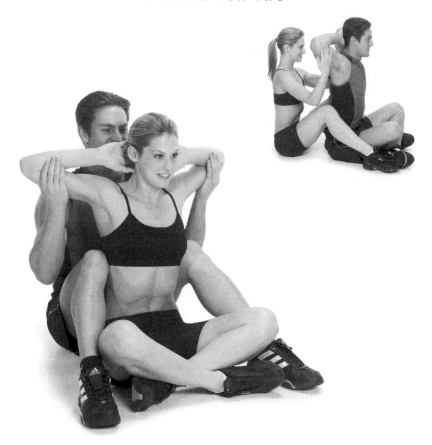

THE BUTTERFLY

Your partner should sit cross-legged on the floor, with her hands behind her head and her elbows out to the sides. You sit behind her, with your legs on either side of hers. Place your hands on her arms just above her elbows. Next, *gently* pull her elbows back toward you, until she feels a stretch across her chest. Don't pull too hard or too fast. Then it's her turn to stretch you. Hold each stretch for 30 seconds. Repeat several times.

▶*Sexual Gains:* **Improves range of motion and comfort when switching from one position to another or when you get adventurous with silk scarves and bedposts.**

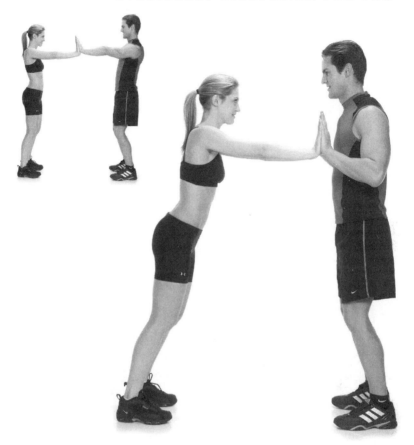

SHOULDER PRESS

Stand face to face with your partner. Your feet should be shoulder-width apart and your knees slightly bent. Extend your arms in front so that your palms touch and your fingers point to the ceiling. Have your partner bend her elbows, easing you toward her. Hold for about 10 seconds, or as long as is comfortable. She then pushes you back to the upright position and leans toward you. Try 10 to 20 times in each direction.

▶*Sexual Gains:* **Stretches the shoulders and arms, allowing each of you to reach down with ease for manual stimulation during foreplay and intercourse.**

CHAPTER 8

THE *BUILT* *FOR SEX* WORKOUT

NEWS FLASH: WOMEN APPRECIATE MEN WITH GOOD PHYSIQUES JUST AS MUCH AS MEN ENJOY FIT WOMEN. IMAGINE THAT.

Men will always be more visually inclined than women, and you can thank your lucky stars for that. Very few of the women we talked to listed Stallone-like muscles at the top of their wish lists. In fact, they're far less likely than men to reject a potential suitor because he's in less-than-perfect shape. But do they appreciate a well-toned body? You bet.

"A muscular upper body and strong arms are a real turn-on," said a 41-year-old hospital administrator in Buffalo. *"I love toned legs, when you can see the outline of his calf and quad muscles,"* said a 33-year-old Portland, Oregon, biologist. And this from a 37-year-old medical student in Albuquerque: *"Some men have a great chest or a nice butt that you just want to get your hands on. But that doesn't mean he has to be 6 feet tall or as strong as an ox."*

If nothing else, it's worth staying in shape—or getting there if you haven't yet made the commitment to buckle down in the gym—just to make yourself more attractive to a current or future partner. The benefits don't stop there. Men who stay in shape have more energy. More energy for sex, for working, for life in general. Exercise makes you happier and more self-assured. Most important, it improves the machinery—bloodflow, nerve activity, and brain chemistry, for example—that you need for full-bore sex appeal and performance.

FIT FOR LOVE

How strong do you have to be for sex? Stronger than you might think—unless your idea of passionate coupling is to imitate one of the stiffs on *Six Feet Under*. Even when you're in the passive, man-on-the-bottom position, you need strong abs and hips to push your body upward. Men who are really out of shape often find themselves getting fatigued before the act is done—as well as sore the next day. That's not very sexy. Or satisfying. And that's an *easy* position. How are you going to feel when you try something more athletic?

If you plan on doing anything more vigorous than just lying there during sex, you're going to need strength, flexibility, and endurance. Consider the man-on-top position. You need a strong chest and strong arms to move with any kind of freedom as well as to hold your weight off your partner. Sex while standing? You'd better have some muscles in your calves, hamstrings, and butt.

"When I'm on top, I find it hard to hold myself up for long periods of time," admits a 21-year-old student in Pittsburgh. *"With all the thrusting and whatnot, my back and abs seem to give out sooner than I'd like."*

The doctors we talked to said that this guy's story is hardly unique. Even though men are more health conscious today than they've ever been, that doesn't always translate into committed workouts. Basically, we spend way too much time at our desks, sitting in our cars, and taking up couch space. Our sex lives are paying the price. Even our *desire* for sex may be heading downhill.

It's not news to exercise physiologists that men who are sedentary can have significant drops in testosterone, the "male" hormone that fuels libido. Add to that the natural drop in testosterone that occurs when men get older, and you can see why a lot of us aren't exactly thrilled with our bedroom oomph.

None of this is inevitable. The amount of exercise that you need for optimal sexual fitness is modest. Half an hour or so in the gym most days of the week will give you endurance, energy, and sex drive that you didn't even know you had. Harder workouts, if you're so inclined, can boost your performance even more. Finnish researchers recently reported that 30-year-old men who engaged in regular weight lifting had significant boosts in testosterone. More testosterone quickly translates to more muscle bulk, faster recovery after workouts, and in some cases, a boost in libido.

"I'm living proof," a 23-year-old student in Boston told us. *"I lost 80 pounds and started lifting. I now have more sex and better sex for longer periods, with no next-day soreness."*

Better sex by itself should be reason enough to strive for the exercise edge. But it's not the only reason.

▶ Men who lift weights get *more* limber, not less. Your balance will improve as well.

▶ Strength training increases bone strength and density. That means less risk of fractures.

▶ It "oils" the joints and lowers the risk of arthritis. It makes it easier to ski, run, or just get around in this world without bum joints.

▶ It increases the level of beneficial HDL cholesterol, which carts the artery-clogging stuff out of your bloodstream before it lays down rock-hard deposits in the arteries that supply the penis.

▶ Men who start a strength-training program invariably report a huge increase in confidence—the quality that nearly all women rate at the top of their sex-appeal charts.

Whether you're interested mainly in building muscle, strengthening bones, or increasing sexual stamina, lifting weights should be your first choice. Muscles grow only in response to high-intensity over-load—pumping iron, in other words. Moving your arms up and

ATHLETES AND ABSTINENCE

When the Los Angeles Dodgers struggled early in the 2003 season, more than a few commentators floated the suggestion that their perfor-mance might improve if players took a little break from their, er, marital arrangements. None of the players actually volunteered (publicly, at least) to "give it up" for the team, and the Dodgers eventually found their footing and made the playoffs anyway.

This story is a perfect illustration of the widespread belief that athletes who have sex before competing somehow lose their edge. The myth persists even though scientific studies—yes, researchers have studied it—clearly show that having sex in no way diminishes an athlete's perfor-mance. One study tested the grip strength of married athletes, ages 24 to 49, the morning after intercourse and the morning after abstinence. There were no differences in grip strength on either morning. A few years later, another study looked at grip strength plus aerobic capacity and coordination. Again, sex the night before made no difference. In fact, some research suggests that athletes actually perform better when they roll in the hay before they play.

down all day won't do a thing for bulk or strength. But put something heavy in your hands, and if that something is heavier than what your arms are accustomed to, you're going to get stronger.

MORE OF WHAT YOU ARE

If you're new to the health-club scene, check your ego at the door. It doesn't matter if you're burly, skinny, tanned, or pale—your physique isn't going to match up to the guys who are clustered around dumbbells the size of Volkswagens. More than a few men walk into the gym and instantly "compare and despair"—and give up because they're too self-conscious to work out next to men who look like they move refrigerators all day.

If you really want to make yourself feel better, remind yourself that (1) a lot of those guys have been lifting for years, (2) the real-life monsters among them have probably been blasting steroids, and (3) all of those black-market drugs are inexorably wrecking them with acne, liver damage, and impotence—and reducing their testicles to the size of peanuts.

Trainers are used to men who come in the door with visions of tree-trunk thighs and anaconda arms filling their heads. Sure, you could be the next Mr. Universe, but that has less to do with commitment than with your basic physical makeup. A strength-training program can make you more of what you already are; it won't transform you into something you're not. A tall, thin man isn't going to emerge a year later with a neck like Mike Tyson's, any more than a short, stocky guy is going to get whippet lean.

And that's a good thing. Research backs up what the women we surveyed said. Yes, they like physical fitness and good muscle tone, but chances are they're looking for a regular guy—not the guy grinning at you from the cover of a body-building magazine. Two studies from the University of Texas in Austin found that women preferred men with waist-to-hip ratios in the normal range. Sure, that means John Goodman wouldn't make their "hotties" list, but neither would Arnold Schwarzenegger.

Lifting weights will definitely improve your health. It will probably boost your libido and your ability to sustain erections. What it won't do is overturn your basic genetic structure. Ever wonder why so many bench-press champs are stubby little guys with short arms? They were born with short bones, which give them great leverage. Anyone who lifts regularly will get bigger and stronger. The extent to which you bulk up has a lot to do with the genes that nature gave you.

Consider your muscle makeup. All men possess a combination of fast-twitch and slow-twitch muscles. Men with a greater percentage of slow-twitch muscles are better suited to aerobic exercise (think distance runners); they'll have a hard time adding much muscle mass. Those with an edge in fast-twitch fibers put on muscle and gain strength more easily—and tend to accumulate body fat more quickly (think power lifters). You can't change your basic muscle equation. The percentage of fast- and slow-twitch fibers that you're born with is the percentage you'll keep.

Age also plays a role in how quickly you'll advance. A man's testosterone levels rise sharply in his second decade of life and continue rising at a slower pace until about age 30. All of that testosterone makes it easy to add muscle mass. Once you're in your 40s, though, you have to work harder to get the same effect.

Researchers in the world of exercise science spend their whole careers studying the finer points of weight lifting. For the most part, though, it pretty much boils down to this: Pick it up, put it down, pick it up again. There isn't a whole lot more to it than that. Of course, there is a handful of training tips that you'll want to keep in mind.

START WITH THE 8-WEEK RULE. If you're just starting out, you'll want to stick with the same basic program—these exercises for your biceps, those for your chest, and so on—for about 8 weeks. That's about how long it takes to kick your muscles into gear and prime your body. It also takes about that long to lock yourself into the habit of exercise.

SHAKE IT UP IN TWO. A lot of experienced lifters find themselves in an exercise rut. They do the same exercises and keep doing them, month after month. There are two problems with this approach. This first is tedium; doing the same exercises again and again is about as exciting as brushing your teeth. More important, muscles need change to keep growing. Sure, you'll keep getting stronger if you do the same workouts, but after about 8 weeks, the gains start to accrue at a snail's pace. You'll get more improvements

I LOVE YOU, SUE . . . ER, CINDY

Plenty of men having sex with one woman fill their heads with fantasies about someone else, and plenty of women do the same. Most of the time, the fantasies never make the injudicious journey from the brain to the mouth—which is a good thing, because no one wants to be called by the wrong name during moments of passion.

Is it a kind of mental infidelity to think of someone else during sex? Some women (and men) think it is. Researchers, on the other hand, say that nearly everyone does it on occasion. In most of these cases, the fantasies that occur during sex are no different from any other fantasies: They can stir your sense of eroticism without ever crossing over into reality.

There is one difference, though. In general, sharing fantasies with your partner can bring the two of you closer, but admitting that you're thinking of someone else altogether probably isn't the smartest thing to do.

Of course, all sorts of things can slip out in the heat of the moment. Which is why more than a few wise lovers never use their partners' names during sex. Generic terms of endearment—"Oh, Baby"—work just as well and minimize the possibility of mistakes.

more quickly if you vary your workouts—adding new exercises, subtracting old ones, or adding twists and refinements—about every 2 weeks. The idea is to avoid training plateaus—those dead zones where further improvement virtually stops.

WORK HARD, REST HARDER. As long as men have been lifting weights, trainers have been arguing about the optimal amount of downtime. These days, the usual advice for regular guys is to lift 3 days a week—every other day, for example—and rest in between. Men in their 20s or 30s who are already in great shape might do better with four weekly workouts. Unless you're a competitive athlete, it's highly unlikely that working out more often will provide extra benefits. If anything, it will increase your risk of injury.

Rest is important for another reason. You might think that your muscles get larger while you're lifting, but that's not what happens. When you're at the gym, you're actually tearing down muscle fibers. The growth phase occurs when muscles repair themselves—and that happens only *after* you leave the gym.

FIND A CLUB THAT WORKS

Most men have tried lifting weights at one time or another. Most have signed up at a health club. And most stick with it—until they find something more interesting to do, like setting up a home entertainment system.

Why do so many good intentions get derailed? Part of it is habit. It takes about 6 weeks before any new activity stops feeling new and becomes just another part of your life, like pulling on your socks every morning. It's also because your whole body rebels when you're out of shape. Start pushing those tired, locked-tight muscles farther than they're used to going, and they're going to fight back. Almost no one enjoys working out for the first week or two. At best, it seems boring—and at worst, it hurts.

You have to push through that initial despair zone. Finding a good club is the best way to do it. Here's what experts advise.

PUT CONVENIENCE FIRST. Just about every city has at least a few health clubs that resemble opulent palaces, replete with fresh towels, the latest glistening chrome, and glass-walled aerobics rooms to facilitate women-watching. They're great places to hang out. They're even great places to work out. But if they aren't located in an area that's near your home or office—or somewhere in between—you'll find all sorts of reasons not to bother. The best gym, even if it's a sweat-stained cave with flickering fluorescent lights that haven't been changed since the Carter Administration, is the one that's easiest to get to.

CHECK OUT THE INVENTORY. Health clubs have taken a hint from big-box shopping centers: warehouse-size spaces with an abundance of benches, free weights, and machines. It's a good approach. Even if you like the cozy atmosphere of an intimate, small-scale club, the last thing you want is to come in all fired up and then spend 20 minutes or so bored out of your nut because clots of muscle-heads won't budge from the machines. Before you sign on the dotted line, drop by the club a few times at the hours you're most likely to go. You should be able to launch into your workout without having to wait more than a few minutes to get to a weight bench or machine.

SCHEDULE A SESSION. Nearly all health clubs offer one or two consultations with a trainer as part of the sign-up cost. Take advantage of it. If you're totally new to lifting, you'll want to get solid instruction on using the equipment, honing your technique, and not getting hurt. Even if you've been lifting for years, a trainer can help correct bad habits and mistakes that you've unconsciously slipped into.

KNOW THE RAP ON REPS. Lifting, like any specialized activity, has its share of jargon. About all you really need to know is the difference between reps and sets.

Rep is short for repetition. If you lift a weight eight consecutive times, you've done eight reps. Sets are groups of repetitions—for example, three sets of eight repetitions.

Once you know that, the rest is mostly details—details that, for the average guy, won't make a whit of difference. It's true that doing multiple sets adds bulk to muscles more quickly than doing single sets. Some trainers swear that you're better off doing a single set of all-out exercises, heaving the maximum weight you can manage. Others argue for doing multiple sets of lesser intensity. Don't worry about it. If your schedule permits, by all means take the time to do multiple sets. If time is short, make do with singles. All of the refinements are mainly for guys who take the whole thing way too seriously. Let's face it, if you haven't done a lot of lifting in the past, any kind of lifting is going to make a difference. You can always refine your workout later.

LIFT FOR TWO, RELAX FOR FOUR. There's no such thing as speed lifting, not that you'd know it from watching the supermacho, muscle-packed dudes who turn every lifting move into something that sounds like a bus smash. They heave up impossibly huge weights, then let them come crashing down. It's all posturing. For one thing, lowering weights too quickly reduces muscle-building strain on the muscles. It's also a great way to get hurt. The fact is, those guys could probably cut the weights in half and get the same or better workouts if they took their time and used good form.

The fastest way to build muscle is to lift and lower weights with total control. The idea is to let your muscles, not gravity, guide each move. You want to complete the exertion phase in a count of two and the relaxing phase in a count of four. Don't obsess over the numbers, though. The most important thing is to lift naturally, without heaving and grunting—or letting go at the end.

KEEP PUSHING. The only way you'll develop bigger, stronger muscles is to work with progressively heavier weights. Once you're able to complete, say, eight repetitions at a given weight, it's time to bump up the weight. Research has shown that beginners usually do best when they start with a weight that's about 40 percent less than the maximum weight they could possibly handle. For example, if you can lift 100 pounds on the bench press when you go all out, start with 60 pounds. Stick with it for a week or two, or until it's clearly too easy. At that point, add more weight.

▼

Men who lift weights regularly tend to have less acne than men who are sedentary. Reason: Sweating heavily during exercise, assuming you clean your skin thoroughly afterward, flushes the pores of acne-causing dirt and debris.

▲

Start with a weight that allows you to do at least 8 reps. Once you can achieve 12 reps with that weight, increase it by about 5 percent. You'll then be doing 8 reps with the slightly heavier weight. Once you've worked up again to 12 reps with the heavier weight, step it up another 5 percent. The idea is to keep increasing, alternately, reps and resistance, so that you continue to achieve results.

The simplest way to figure out how much weight you should attempt on each exercise is through trial by ordeal. Pick up a weight and try eight reps. If you can't make eight, you need to select a lighter weight. Keep going until you've found a weight you can lift eight times, but not nine. The ideal weight should fatigue you by rep five but not actually wear you out until eight.

If your main goal is to improve cardiovascular endurance, you'll want to focus on doing more repetitions with lighter weights. For brute strength, you'll employ heavier weights in fewer repetitions. For overall muscle tone—the optimal place for beginners—lift medium weights, trying to complete 10 to 12 repetitions per set.

SPLIT YOUR ROUTINES. This simply means working different muscle groups on different days. Many lifters, for example, work their chests and backs on one day, then their legs and arms on the next. The advantage of this approach is that you get a more concentrated workout. At the same time, each muscle group gets a day off when you shift your focus to a different area. Over the course of two or three workouts, you hit all of your muscles—and then you start all over again.

You can split a routine in any number of ways.

▶ Divide your workouts into upper- and lower-body routines.

▶ Divide them into pushing and pulling exercises. Pushing exercises include squats and presses, while pulling movements include deadlifts, curls, rows, and pulldowns.

▶ Divide your body front to back. Most of the muscles on the front of your body, along with your calves and triceps, involve pushing exercises. The muscles on the back of your body, along with the biceps, usually involve pulling movements.

▶ Work the big muscles first. Time is limited. Energy is limited. And let's face it, your patience has limits as well. There will always be times when you drag yourself to the gym, do one or two sets of a few exercises, then make a sudden detour to the hot tub. To ensure that you can get some sort of workout every time you go, focus on the big muscles first: the thighs, chest, and so on. Save the small-muscle workouts, like those focusing on the wrists or triceps, for the last part of the workout. Even if you bail early, the big-muscle exercises will have hit most of the minor muscles as well.

SEX-SPECIFIC STRENGTH TRAINING

There are all sorts of reasons men lift weights. The main ones are to look better and feel better, and that's about as good as motivation gets. But in the following pages, we've done something a little different. We talked to the country's top trainers and asked them to help us design a workout plan devoted entirely to better sex.

It's true that *any* weight lifting plan will go a long way toward boosting the endurance and strength that you need for good sex, but most of the exercise you get in the bedroom brings specific muscle groups into play. When you tone and strengthen these muscles, you'll find that you'll be able to have sex longer than you did before. You'll have more energy. You'll be able to hold yourself in the most common sexual positions without fatigue.

This program is simple, yet it hits every major muscle group. It's divided into two phases. Phase 1 concentrates on building your strength base. Even if you do nothing else, it will give you strength and flexibility in places you never had them—and you (and your partner) will notice the difference within a few weeks, in bed and out.

Once you've mastered the exercises in Phase 1—for most men, it will take several months, although some of you might be ready after 4 to 6 weeks—it's time to concentrate on specific muscles. Narrowing your focus to specific muscles will tone and sculpt your body, while at the same time improving your strength and endurance when the lights go down.

What about the "Position of Strength" exercises you see at the end of this chapter? How do those fit into the plan? The most effective way to incorporate those into your workouts is to prioritize them by starting each workout with one or two of the exercises.

As you'll see in the charts after each workout, this program requires working out 4 days a week. We've divided the charts into "Day One" and "Day Two" workouts, each of which will be repeated twice a week, giving you time off in between.

As for equipment, you'll need either access to a gym or a nicely appointed home setup. If you don't have either, do the at-home variations. All you'll need are some water bottles; soup cans; and heavy boxes, suitcases, sandbags, or cinder blocks. Or you might consider buying a set of dumbbells and some resistance bands. All told, they won't cost nearly as much as a home gym or gym membership.

PHASE **1**

LOWER BODY ▶

THIS IS THE PLACE TO START FOR BETTER SEX. The most powerful muscles in your body are in the lower body. It makes sense because just about every position you find yourself in, sexual or otherwise, puts at least some strain on the legs, hips, and butt. These are also the muscles that give the power and strength to maintain and change sexual positions.

PHASE **1**: LOWER BODY

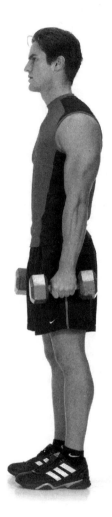

DUMBBELL LUNGE

START: Grab a dumbbell in each hand, with your palms facing your body, and stand with your feet hip-width apart.

FINISH: Keeping your back straight, take a long step forward with your right leg. Bend your leg until your right thigh is parallel with the floor. Your left leg should be extended, with your knee slightly bent and almost touching the floor. Keep your right foot stationary as you straighten your right leg. Switch legs and repeat on the other side.

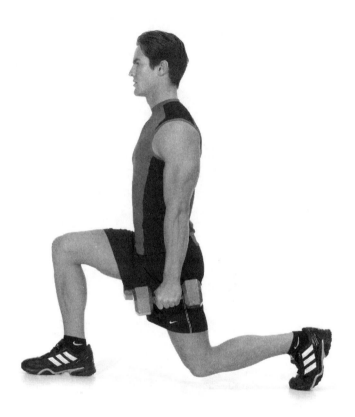

AT-HOME VARIATION: Substitute full plastic water or detergent bottles or unopened soup cans, depending on how heavy you want the weight to be. (Not pictured.)

▶*Sexual Gains:* **This exercise works the butt and the front of the thigh, while putting little stress on the knee. It also strengthens the hamstrings, improves balance and posture, and supports missionary, standing, and kneeling positions.**

PHASE **1**: LOWER BODY

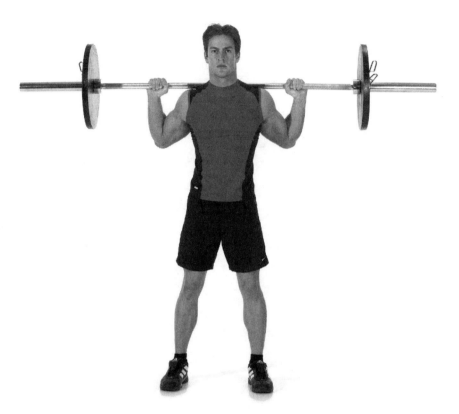

BARBELL SQUAT

START: Place a barbell at shoulder level on a squat rack. Grip the bar with your hands slightly more than shoulder-width apart, palms facing front. Step under the bar so that it's evenly positioned across your upper back and shoulders, not your neck. Stand up straight with your feet hip-width apart and your knees slightly bent. Don't drop your head; keep it in line with your torso.

FINISH: Keeping your feet flat and torso straight, bend your knees slightly and squat down as though sitting in a chair behind you. Don't allow your knees to extend past your toes. Continue moving downward until your thighs are parallel with the floor. Then slowly rise to a standing position.

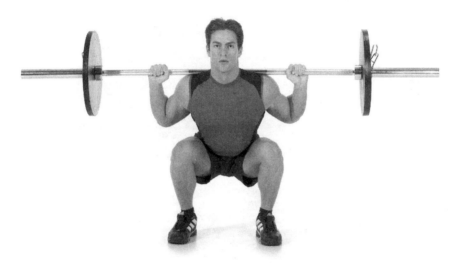

AT-HOME VARIATION: Wall Squat (page 220)

▶*Sexual Gains:* **All told, the squat works more than 200 different muscles. It is the main exercise used by elite athletes for strengthening the large muscle groups—specifically, the front thigh (quadriceps), butt, and hamstrings. It also works the calves and shins, along with muscles in the shoulders, arms, and back. Great for standing and athletic positions.**

PHASE 1: LOWER BODY

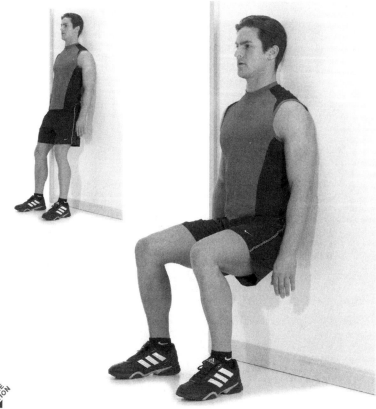

AT-HOME VARIATION

WALL SQUAT

START: Stand with your back flat against a wall, with your feet a little wider than shoulder-width apart and your toes pointed slightly outward. Bend at your knees, keeping your weight centered over your feet.

FINISH: Lower your body as resistance, until your knees are bent 90 degrees. Straighten up slowly, concentrating on using your legs to slide up the wall. *Note:* Holding a heavy object—a couple of filled water bottles, for example—will give you more resistance.

PHASE 1

UPPER BODY ▶

JUST AS YOU CAN'T HAVE GOOD SEX WITHOUT A STRONG LOWER BODY, YOU CAN'T HOPE TO PERFORM AT YOUR BEST UNLESS YOUR BACK, CHEST, AND ARMS ARE EQUALLY STRONG. It's especially important to work the back, an area men tend to neglect. When properly strengthened and defined, the muscles give the back a visually pleasing V shape, which has the added benefit of making your waist look smaller.

PHASE **1**: UPPER BODY

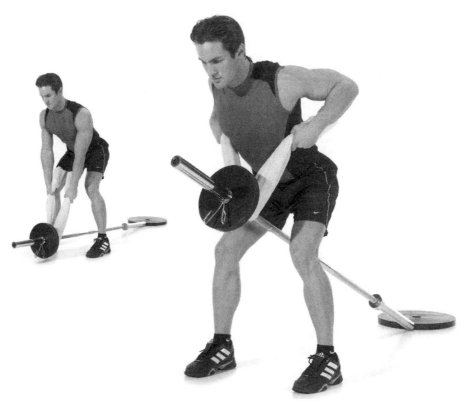

BENT-OVER ROW

START: Using an Olympic-size (45-pound) bar, wedge one end in a corner and place a 25-pound or lighter weight plate on the other end. Wrap a towel around the bar, just under the weight plate. Straddle the bar, keeping your knees slightly bent. Your chin should be up, your chest out, stomach in, shoulders back, and back flat.

FINISH: Pull the bar to your chest, slightly arching your back and letting your elbows rise above your chest. Slowly lower the bar to arm's length, then repeat.

AT-HOME VARIATION: Suitcase Row (opposite)

▶*Sexual Gains:* Improves posture and form and is particularly important for vigorous sex, which tends to put a lot of pressure on the lower back.

PHASE **1**: UPPER BODY

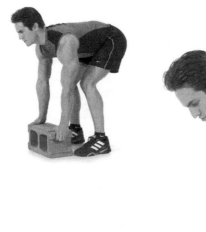

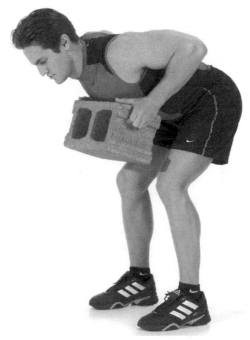

AT-HOME VARIATION

SUITCASE ROW

START: Set a full suitcase (or sandbag, cinder block, railroad tie, whatever) in front of you. Stand with your legs comfortably apart, then bend over at your hips, with your knees bent and your back flat, and grab the sides of the bag.

FINISH: Use your back and biceps to pull the suitcase up to your chest, keeping it close to your body. Pause, then slowly return to the starting position.

PHASE 1: UPPER BODY

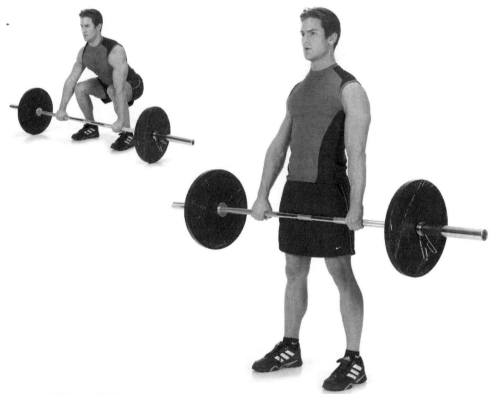

DEADLIFT

START: Load a barbell and set it on the floor. Squat behind it with your feet shoulder-width apart. Grab it overhand, with your hands just outside your legs, your shoulders over or just behind the bar, your arms straight, and your back flat or slightly arched.

FINISH: Straighten up, lifting the weight to a standing position. Push with your heels and pull the weight to your body as you stand. Pause, then slowly return to the starting position.

AT-HOME VARIATION: Boxlift (opposite)

▶*Sexual Gains:* This is another superb exercise for strengthening all of the major back muscles, important for energetic sex. Be sure to do this exercise slowly. You defeat its purpose if you use momentum to finish your reps.

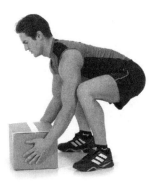

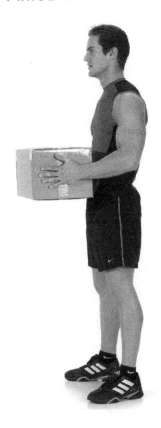

BOXLIFT

START: Set a weighted box on the floor. Stand behind the box, with your feet shoulder-width apart and your toes pointed out slightly. Squat behind the box and grab it with a neutral grip (palms facing each other).

FINISH: Straighten up, lifting the box to a standing position. Push with your heels and pull the weight to your body as you stand. Pause, then slowly return to the starting position.

PHASE 1: UPPER BODY

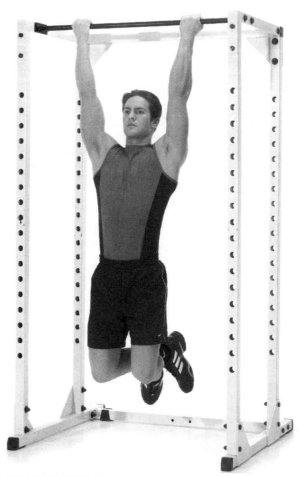

CHINUP (SUPINATED)

START: Using an underhand grip, grab a chinup bar and place your hands shoulder-width apart. Hang from the bar with your elbows slightly bent and your ankles crossed.

FINISH: Slowly pull yourself up until your chin is over the bar. Hold for a second or two, then slowly return to the starting position.

AT-HOME VARIATION: At-home variations for Chinups are not really practical. You're much better off purchasing a chinup bar.

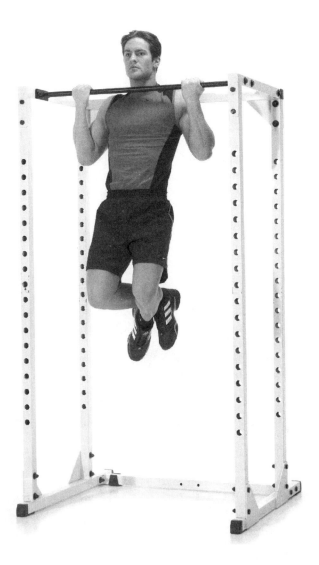

▶*Sexual Gains:* Chinups look easy, but they require you to raise your entire body weight. They work all of the major upper- and mid-body muscles, including those in the back, chest, and arms. You need a strong back and chest to support yourself in the man-on-top position. Your partner will get a visual treat because most women are attracted to a well-developed chest.

PHASE 1: UPPER BODY

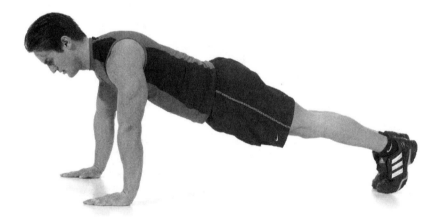

PUSHUP

START: Support your body on the balls of your feet and your hands, positioning the latter slightly wider than shoulder-width apart, palms flat on the floor. Keep your eyes on the floor and your legs, back, and neck in a straight line.

FINISH: Lower your torso until your chest almost touches the floor, then slowly return to the starting position.

TO WORK YOUR CHEST MORE: Place your hands more than shoulder-width apart.

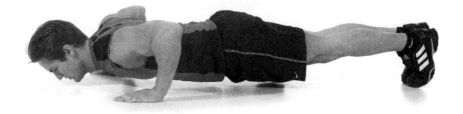

TO WORK YOUR BACK AND ARMS MORE: Place your hands together underneath your chest, thumbs and index fingers touching.

AT-HOME VARIATION: Not necessary. You can do Pushups anywhere, anytime.

▶*Sexual Gains:* **Besides supporting you in the man-on-top position and all its variations, a strong chest and arms are required for standing positions in which you lift your partner off the floor.**

PHASE **1**: UPPER BODY

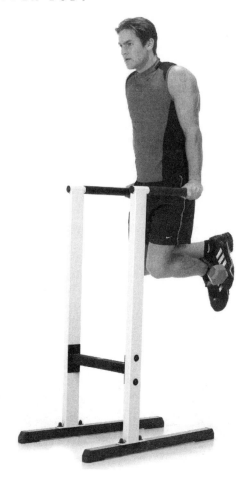

DIP

START: Using the parallel bars or dip station at the gym, grab the handles with a neutral grip. Jump up and steady yourself. Start the movement with your arms straight but not locked and your body perfectly still. You can cross your legs behind you or leave them hanging straight down. The more upright you are, the harder you work your triceps. Leaning forward shifts the work to your chest and shoulders.

FINISH: Slowly lower your body until your upper arms are parallel with the floor. Push back up to the starting position. You can make

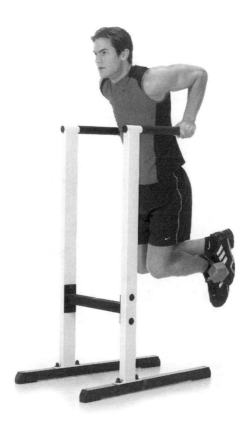

the move harder by wearing a weighted dip belt or clenching a dumbbell between your ankles.

AT-HOME VARIATION: Table Dip (page 232)

▶*Sexual Gains:* **Dips build a strong chest, arms, and shoulders. Specifically, they work the deltoid muscles in your shoulders. They're the key to moving your arms, and they play a central role in many sexual positions, including man on top. Surprisingly, your shoulder muscles come into play when you're performing oral sex if you're propped up on your elbows.**

PHASE 1: UPPER BODY

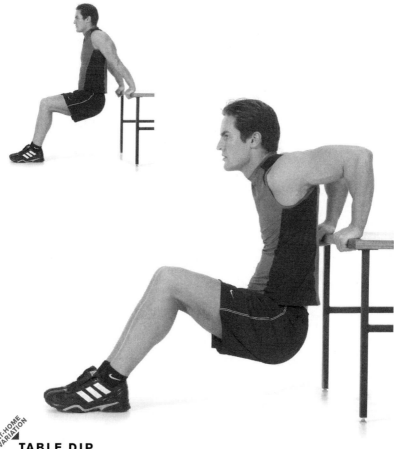

AT-HOME
VARIATION

TABLE DIP

START: Position your hands shoulder-width apart on a secure table, palms down. Walk your feet out so that your knees form a 90-degree angle.

FINISH: Lower your torso until your butt is within an inch of the floor. Slowly return to the starting position.

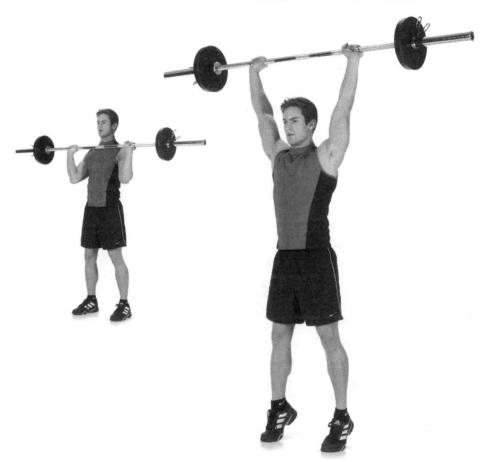

BARBELL PUSH PRESS

START: Balance a barbell on the fronts of your shoulders, with your hands shoulder-width apart and your elbows pointed up. Your knees should be slightly bent.

FINISH: Push the bar straight up until your elbows are almost locked. At the same time, rise slightly on your toes. Then slowly return to the starting position.

AT-HOME VARIATION: Anterior Pushup (page 234)

▶*Sexual Gains:* **Another great exercise for increasing the shoulder strength you need for man-on-top positions.**

PHASE **1**: UPPER BODY

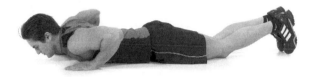

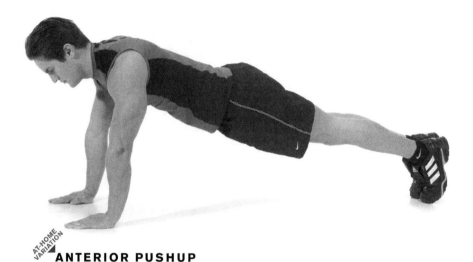

AT-HOME VARIATION

ANTERIOR PUSHUP

START: Lie facedown on the floor, with your hands flat under your shoulders and your toes touching the floor.

FINISH: Push off the floor by extending your arms, keeping your body and legs stiff. Use only your palms and toes to hold your body up. While in the arms-extended position, round your back (this will add another inch off the floor). Finally, retract your shoulder blades, then bend your arms slowly, lowering your chest until it just barely touches the floor. Push back up again and repeat.

▶*Sexual Gains:* **A variation of the Barbell Push Press, this is another great exercise for increasing shoulder strength.**

ABDOMINALS ▶

THE ABDOMINAL MUSCLES ARE WHAT ALLOW YOU TO BEND FORWARD, BACKWARD, AND SIDE TO SIDE. Sexually, they're the muscles that provide strong thrusting power, while at the same time allowing you to subtly alter your position and angle of thrust.

Of course, to take best advantage of your abs, you should first lose your gut. *"My sex life is better now that my gut isn't in the way for either of us,"* says a 58-year-old retired high school principal who embarked on a weight-loss plan along with an ab-strengthening workout.

Once the gut starts to go, you'll notice that there is quite a number of muscles hidden away in there. The major ones include the transversus abdominis, which helps keep the abdominal wall tight and allows you to maintain a firm erection and control premature ejaculation. The quadratis lumborum are muscles that allow you to bend to each side. The rectus abdominis, or six-pack muscle, is the large, flat muscle running the length of the abdomen that promotes trunk flexion. The external abdominal obliques are muscles that run down the sides and front of the abdomen and allow your body to rotate and bend from side to side. The internal abdominal obliques also enable sideways movements.

Working on all these muscles has clear sexual benefits. *"I've definitely noticed increased endurance, ability, and range of motion through increases in core strength,"* a 29-year-old computer programmer told us.

PHASE **1**: ABDOMINALS

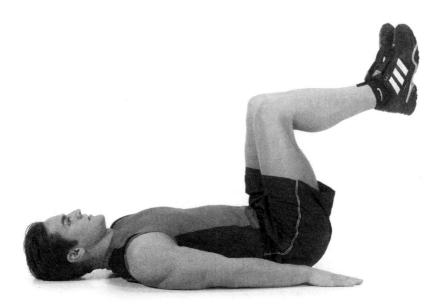

REVERSE CRUNCH

START: Lie on your back, with your arms by your sides. Hold your legs off the floor with your knees bent at a 90-degree angle so your thighs point straight up and your lower legs point straight ahead, parallel with the floor.

FINISH: Roll your pelvis backward and raise your hips a few inches off the floor; your knees should be over your chest. Hold for a moment, then return to the starting position.

AT-HOME VARIATION: Not necessary. You can do most ab exercises anywhere, anytime.

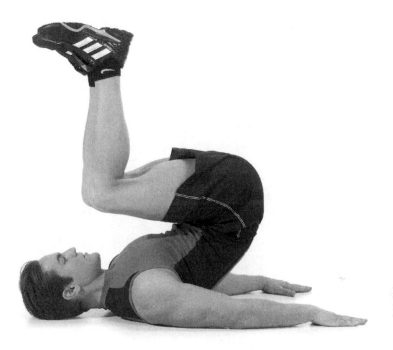

▶*Sexual Gains:* This is among the best exercises for strengthening the lower abdominals, and it's among the easiest. It improves your thrusting endurance and fine-tunes subtle thrusting movements.

PHASE **1**: ABDOMINALS

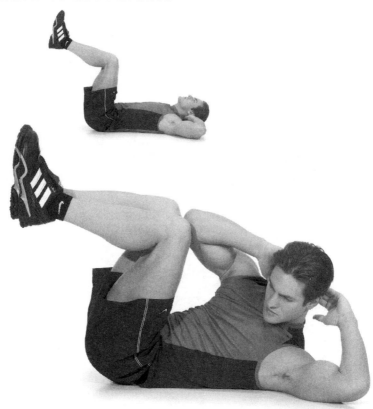

TWISTING OBLIQUE CRUNCH

START: Lie on your back, with your hands loosely touching the back of your head or neck. Bend your knees at a 90-degree angle.

FINISH: Lift your upper body off the floor and twist to the left, until your right elbow touches your left knee. Slowly return to the starting position, then repeat in the opposite direction.

AT-HOME VARIATION: Not necessary.

▶*Sexual Gains:* This exercise strengthens your obliques and is good for side-by-side positions in which you enter your partner from behind and reach around her to stimulate her clitoris. You also use your obliques anytime you attempt some of the more acrobatic positions.

PHASE **1**: ABDOMINALS

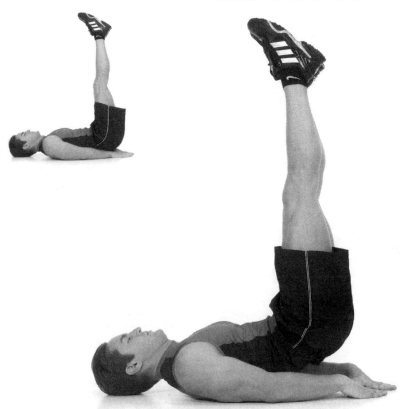

PULSE-UP

START: Lie with your hands flat underneath your tailbone and your legs pointed straight up toward the ceiling, perpendicular to your torso.

FINISH: Pull your navel inward and flex your glutes as you lift your hips just a few inches off the floor. Then lower your hips.

AT-HOME VARIATION: Not necessary.

▶*Sexual Gains:* **Good for thrusting endurance and subtle thrusting movements.**

PHASE 1
WORKOUT PLAN

It's a good idea to warm up before launching into any strength-training workout. Walk briskly, or ride an exercise bike for at least 5 to 10 minutes. It's also a good idea to stretch when the workout is done. See chapter 7 for a complete guide to stretching.

DAY ONE

EXERCISE	SETS	REPS	REP SPEED (SECONDS)	REST INTERVAL
Chinup (supinated)	2	10–12	2 down, 3 up	1 min.
Barbell Squat	2	10–12	2 down, 3 up	1 min.
Pushup	2	10–12	2 down, 3 up	1 min.
Deadlift	2	10–12	2 down, 3 up	2 min.
Pulse-Up	2	10–12	hold 3 at top	10 sec.
Reverse Crunch	2	10–12	2 down, 3 up	1½ min.

DAY TWO

EXERCISE	SETS	REPS	REP SPEED (SECONDS)	REST INTERVAL
Barbell Push Press	2	10–12	3 down, explode up	1 min.
Dumbbell Lunge	2	10–12	2 down, explode up	1 min.
Dip	2	10–12	2 down, 3 up	1 min.
Bent-Over Row	2	10–12	2 down, 3 up	2 min.
Twisting Oblique Crunch	2	10–12	2 down, 2 up	1 min.

PHASE **2**

LOWER BODY ▶

ONCE YOU'VE MASTERED THE EXERCISES IN PHASE 1, WHICH FOR MOST MEN WILL TAKE SEVERAL MONTHS, MOVE ON TO PHASE 2. Here's where you'll start concentrating on specific muscles. As in phase 1, phase 2 has lower body, upper body, and abdominals sections, along with a biceps and triceps section.

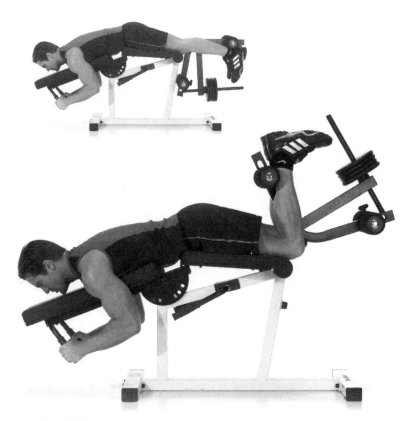

LEG CURL

START: Lie facedown on a leg-curl machine.

FINISH: With your hips flat against the bench and your abdominal muscles tight, curl your legs behind you until your feet are about perpendicular to the bench. Pause, then lower your legs slowly to the starting position, stopping just before your knees are straight.

AT-HOME VARIATION: Dumbbell Leg Curl (opposite)

▶*Sexual Gains:* **Strong hamstrings are essential for standing and kneeling positions.**

PHASE 2: LOWER BODY

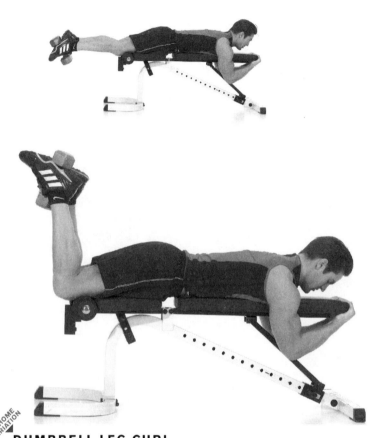

DUMBBELL LEG CURL

START: Set a dumbbell between the insteps of your feet and lie facedown on a flat bench. (This is tricky at first, and you might need someone to help you.) Grab the front or sides of the bench for support.

FINISH: Keeping your hips against the bench, curl the weight up toward your butt. Stop when your lower legs point straight up, then, without pausing, lower the weight slowly.

PHASE 2: LOWER BODY

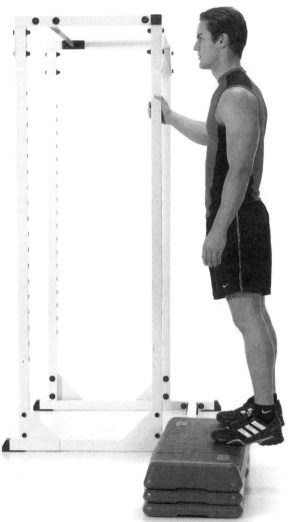

CALF RAISE

START: Stand with the balls of your feet on the edge of a step, with your legs about 12 inches apart. Hold onto the banister or wall for stability.

FINISH: Slowly rise on your toes as far as you can go, hold for a second, then lower yourself back. To work different portions of the calves, shift your feet so that your toes point either in or out.

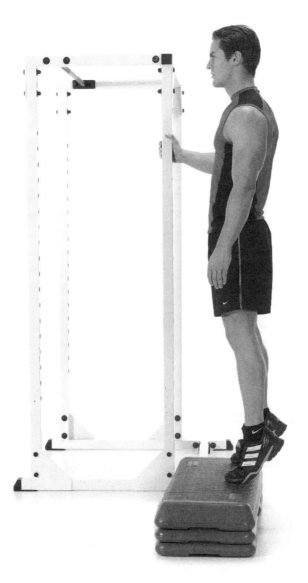

AT-HOME VARIATION: Not necessary.

▶*Sexual Gains:* **Strong calves improve your endurance and strength for standing positions.**

PHASE 2: UPPER BODY

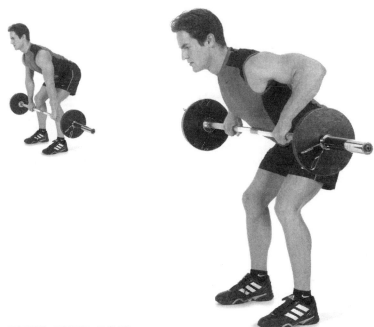

BENT-OVER ROW

START: Stand with your feet shoulder-width apart and your knees bent 15 to 30 degrees. Keep your torso straight, with a slight arch in your back, as you lean forward at the hips. Try to get your torso close to parallel with the floor. Grab the barbell off the floor with a full overhand grip (thumbs wrapped around the bar) that's slightly wider than shoulder width. Let the bar hang at arm's length in front of you.

FINISH: Retract your shoulder blades to start pulling the bar up to the lower part of your sternum (breastbone). Pause at the top, with your chest sticking out toward the bar. Slowly return to the starting position. Try to keep your torso in the same position throughout the movement.

AT-HOME VARIATION: Suitcase Row (opposite)

▶ *Sexual Gains:* **Good for strengthening and sculpting the lower and middle portions of the back. Again, a strong back is essential for standing or kneeling positions and important for stamina during any vigorous lovemaking session.**

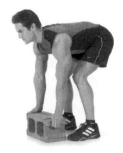

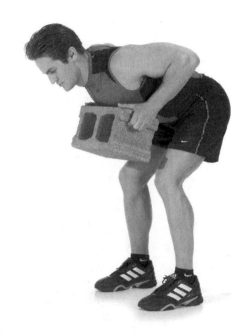

SUITCASE ROW

START: Set a full suitcase (or sandbag, cinder block, railroad tie, whatever) in front of you. Stand with your legs comfortably apart, then bend over at your hips, with your knees bent and your back flat, and grab the sides of the bag.

FINISH: Use your back and biceps to pull the suitcase up to your chest, keeping it close to your body. Pause, then slowly return to the starting position.

PHASE **2**: UPPER BODY

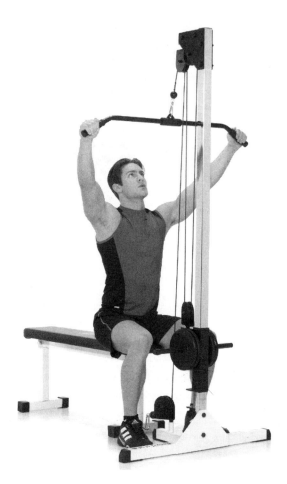

LATERAL PULLDOWN

START: Sit at a lat pulldown machine. Grasp the bar with your hands about shoulder-width apart and a false overhand grip (thumbs on the same side of the bar as your fingers). Your arms should be fully extended overhead and your torso upright or leaning back slightly.

FINISH: Pull the bar straight down until it almost touches your upper chest, while squeezing your shoulder blades together. Slowly return to the starting position with your chest out, keeping full control of the bar at all times.

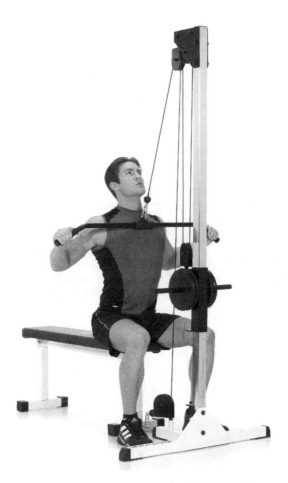

AT-HOME VARIATION: Dumbbell Pullover (page 250)

▶*Sexual Gains:* This exercise works the upper part of
the back, along with the shoulders and arms. It's another great
exercise for man-on-top positions and standing positions in
which you lift your partner off the floor.

PHASE **2**: UPPER BODY

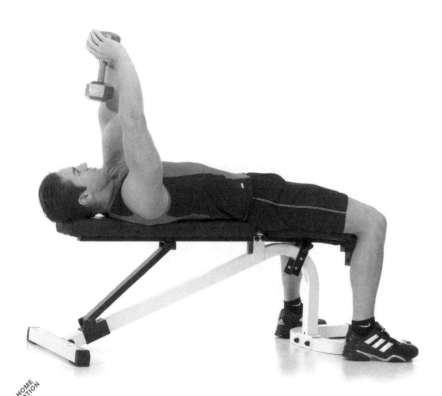

AT-HOME VARIATION

DUMBBELL PULLOVER

START: Lie flat on a bench. Press your head, torso, lower back, and glutes firmly against the surface. Your feet should be flat on the floor (or, if you prefer, the end of the bench). Place one hand around the handle of a dumbbell, then wrap the other over the gripping hand. Extend your arms directly above your collarbone, holding the dumbbell perpendicular to the floor.

FINISH: Keeping your back flat against the bench to elongate your lats, slowly lower the weight behind your head until your arms are in

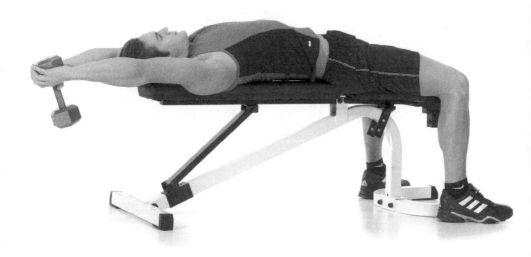

line with your ears. Pause, then pull the weight back up. Slightly bend your elbows throughout.

▶*Sexual Gains:* **This exercise is a variation of the Lateral Pulldown that can be done at home. It works the upper part of the back, along with the shoulders and arms.**

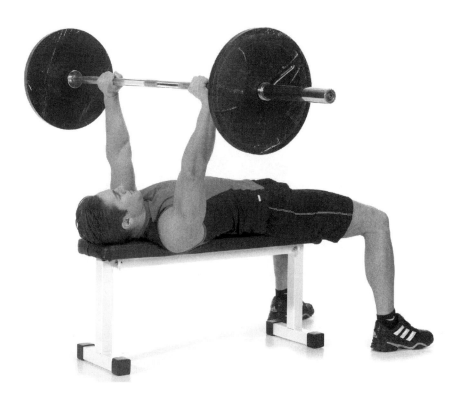

BENCH PRESS

START: Lie flat on a bench, with your feet flat on the floor and your head positioned about eye level under the bar. Grab the barbell with a full overhand grip (thumbs wrapped around the bar), placing your hands about shoulder-width apart. Remove the bar from the uprights and hold it with straight arms over your collarbone. Pull your shoulder blades together in back.

FINISH: Lower the bar, slowly and in control, to just above your nipples. Then press it up and slightly back so it finishes above your

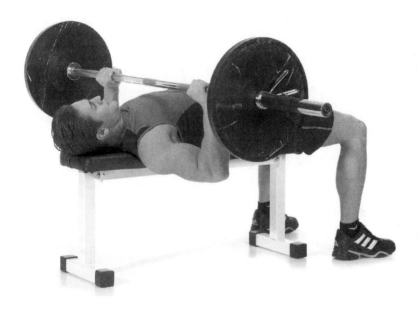

collarbone again. Stop just short of locking your elbows, and keep your shoulder blades pulled back.

AT-HOME VARIATION: Use dumbbells, filled water bottles, or unopened soup cans. (Not pictured.)

▶*Sexual Gains:* **The Bench Press is the main exercise for building a bigger chest, which not only looks great when you're on top but also helps hold you up.**

PHASE 2: UPPER BODY

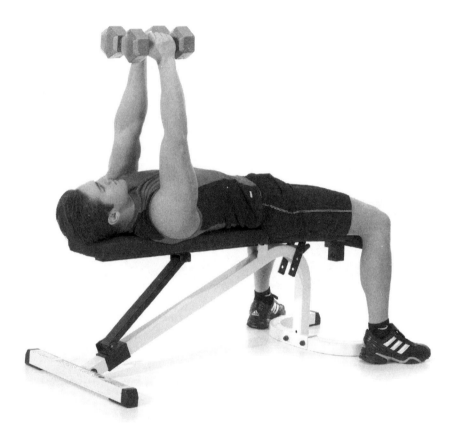

DUMBBELL FLY

START: Grab a pair of dumbbells that are lighter than those you'd use for a dumbbell bench press. Lie flat on a bench, with your feet flat on the floor and the dumbbells at arm's length above your chest.

FINISH: Maintaining a slight bend in your elbows, lower the dumbbells down and back until your upper arms are parallel with the floor and in line with your ears. Pause for a moment, then use your chest to pull the weights back to the starting position, repeating your movements in reverse. Keep your shoulder blades

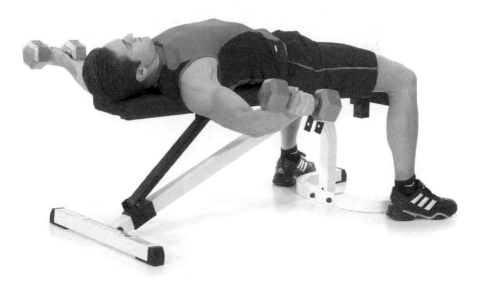

pulled toward each other throughout, and flex your pecs at the top of the movement.

AT-HOME VARIATION: Substitute unopened soup cans or filled water bottles for the dumbbells. (Not pictured.)

▶*Sexual Gains:* **This is similar to the Bench Press, except you have to balance the dumbbells separately—which works your chest muscles even more.**

PHASE **2**: UPPER BODY

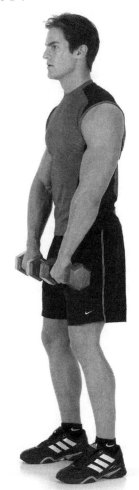

DUMBBELL FRONT RAISE

START: Grab a dumbbell in each hand, with your arms hanging
in front of your thighs. Stand with your feet shoulder-width apart,
knees slightly bent, and lean forward very slightly at the hips (to
avoid leaning back as you lift).

FINISH: Bend your elbows slightly and raise the dumbbells straight
in front of you until your arms are parallel with the floor. Pause, then
slowly return to the starting position.

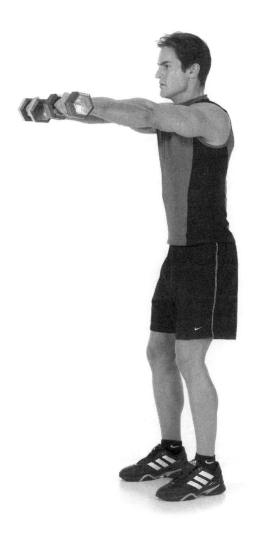

AT-HOME VARIATION: Substitute unopened soup cans or filled water bottles for the dumbbells. (Not pictured.)

▶ *Sexual Gains:* This exercise puts power and definition in your shoulders—and you get an extra workout because you have to balance the dumbbells separately. It's especially good for when you're in the man-on-top position for an extended period of time.

PHASE **2**: UPPER BODY

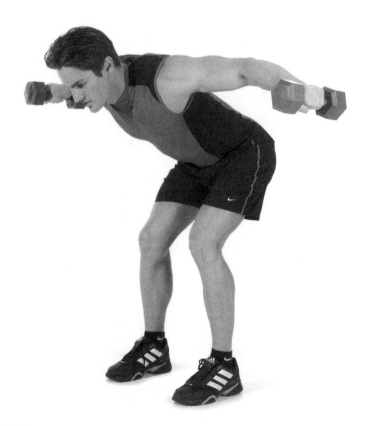

BENT-OVER LATERAL RAISE

START: Sit or stand, with your torso bent forward almost parallel with the floor and your knees slightly spread. Grab a dumbbell in each hand with your palms facing inward, elbows slightly bent.

FINISH: Slowly raise the dumbbells out to your sides, keeping your elbows bent, your back straight, and your head in a neutral position. Squeeze your shoulder blades together at the highest point in the movement. Pause, then slowly lower the dumbbells to the starting position.

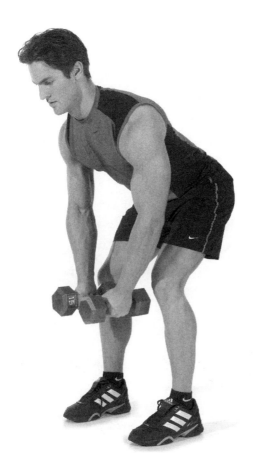

AT-HOME VARIATION: Substitute unopened soup cans or filled water bottles for the dumbbells. (Not pictured.)

▶ *Sexual Gains:* This exercise hits the shoulders at a slightly different angle than the Front Raise, giving you that much extra man-on-top staying power. This exercise is also good for strengthening the muscles that support your neck when you're performing oral sex.

PHASE **2**: BICEPS AND TRICEPS

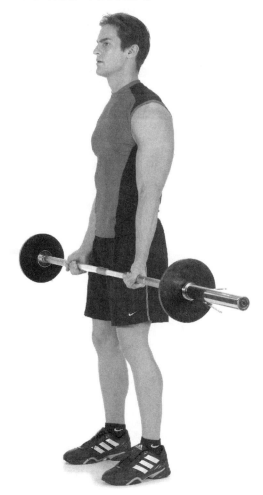

BICEPS CURL

START: Holding a barbell or dumbbells with an underhand grip, stand with your feet shoulder-width apart and your arms down at your sides.

FINISH: Curl your arms up toward your shoulders. Stop and squeeze when the weight is 6 to 8 inches from your shoulders. Keep your abdomen tight, your elbows still, and your upper body straight. Pause, then lower the weight to the starting position.

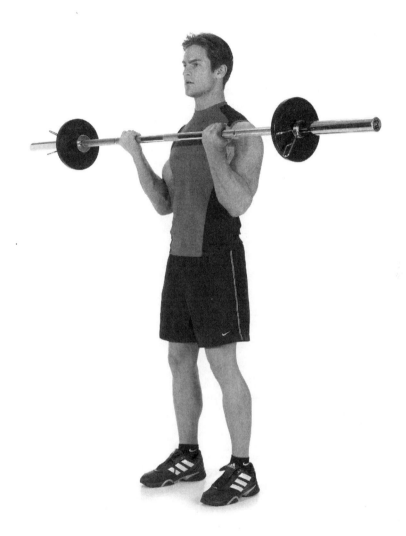

AT-HOME VARIATION: Substitute unopened soup cans or filled water bottles for the barbell or dumbbells. (Not pictured.)

▶*Sexual Gains:* **Strong biceps are necessary for lifting your partner, man-on-top positions, and rear-entry positions in which you support yourself with your arms.**

PHASE 2: BICEPS AND TRICEPS

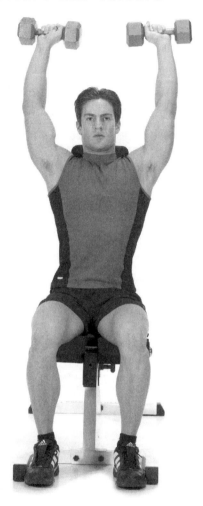

SEATED DUMBBELL TRICEPS EXTENSION

START: Sit on a bench with a 90-degree back support. With a neutral, shoulder-width grip, grab a pair of dumbbells and hold them straight up over your head with your elbows unlocked.

FINISH: Bend at the elbows as you lower the weights down to the sides of your head. Keep your upper arms in the same position and pause when your elbows are bent just past 90 degrees. Return to the starting position.

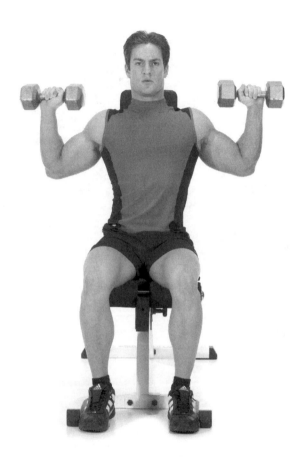

AT-HOME VARIATION: Use filled water bottles or unopened soup cans. (Not pictured.)

▶*Sexual Gains:* Triceps are harder to build than biceps, but you need balanced strength in your arms for maximum muscle power for lifting your partner, man-on-top, and rear-entry positions.

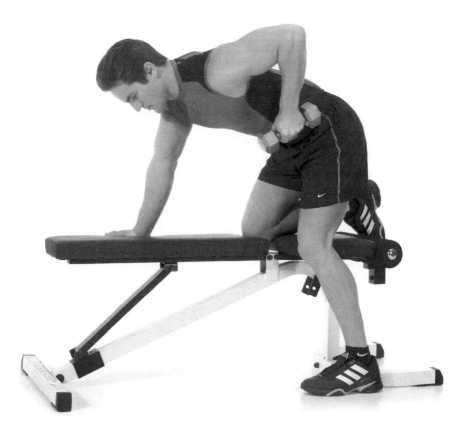

TRICEPS KICKBACK

START: Grab a light dumbbell in your left hand and place your right hand and knee on a bench. Plant your left foot on the floor. Bend forward at the hips so your torso is parallel with the floor. Hold the dumbbell at your side with a neutral grip, elbow pointed toward the ceiling.

FINISH: Lift the weight up and back until your arm is straight. Keep your elbow pointed toward the ceiling and the rest of your body steady. Pause for 2 full seconds, then slowly return to the starting position. Finish the set on the left side before repeating on the right.

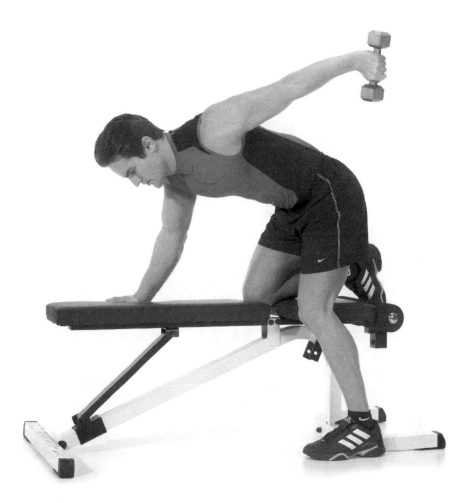

AT-HOME VARIATION: Substitute unopened soup cans or filled water bottles for the dumbbells. (Not pictured.)

▶*Sexual Gains:* Besides needing strong arms to lift your partner or support yourself when you're on top, you also need them during foreplay. You can stimulate your partner manually for much longer if your arms don't get tired.

PHASE 2: ABDOMINALS

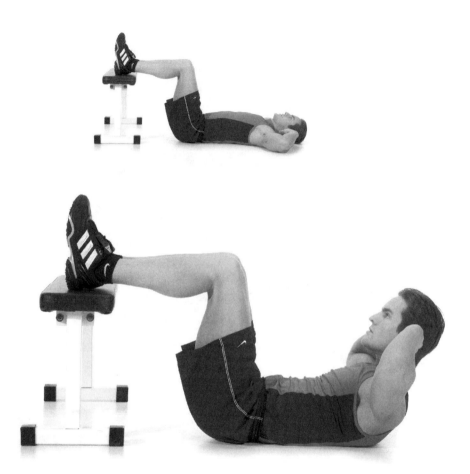

CRUNCH

START: Lie on your back, with your knees bent at 90 degrees or resting on a bench. Hold your hands behind your ears.

FINISH: Use your abs to curl your torso upward 4 to 6 inches, keeping your lower back firmly pressed to the floor. Pause, then slowly lower your back to the floor.

AT-HOME VARIATION: Not necessary.

▶*Sexual Gains:* **This is the core exercise for building strong abs. Two words: Thrusting power.**

PHASE 2: ABDOMINALS

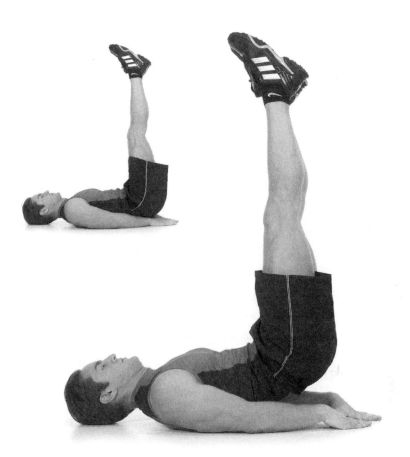

PULSE-UP

START: Lie with your hands underneath your tailbone and your legs pointed straight up toward the ceiling, perpendicular to your torso.

FINISH: Pull your navel inward and flex your glutes as you lift your hips just a few inches off the floor. Then lower your hips.

AT-HOME VARIATION: Not necessary.

▶*Sexual Gains:* **Good for thrusting endurance and subtle thrusting movements.**

PHASE 2
WORKOUT PLAN

Because this phase of the sexual fitness plan is more vigorous than the first, don't rush into it. Work your way through Phase 1 until your muscles no longer feel sore from lactic acid buildup after a workout, roughly 4 to 6 weeks after you start Phase 1.

Phase 2 is divided into push and pull days. On push days, work your chest, shoulders, and triceps—with exercises in which you push the weight. On pull days, work your back and biceps—with exercises that pull weight. Do the lower-body exercises on the second day. Plan on doing the abdominal exercises toward the end of each workout.

Don't be afraid to shuffle the exercises. Varying your workout every few weeks will hit muscles from different angles and with varying degrees of intensity, providing new stimuli ideal for optimal muscle growth. If you're satisfied with the strength and size of your arms, for example, substitute a couple of extra leg or abdominal exercises. Or maybe you're just not getting the results you need from the reverse crunch. Replace it with regular abdominal crunches.

DAY ONE (PUSH)

EXERCISE	SETS	REPS	REP SPEED (SECONDS)	REST INTERVAL
Bench Press	2	10–12	2 down, 3 up	1 min.
Bent-Over Lateral Raise	2	10–12	2 down, 3 up	1 min.
Dip	2	10–12	2 down, 3 up	1 min.
Seated Dumbbell Triceps Ext.	2	10–12	2 down, 3 up	1 min.
Dumbbell Front Raise	2	10–12	2 down, 3 up	1 min.
Triceps Kickback	2	10–12	2 down, 3 up	1 min.
Crunch	2	10–12	hold 3 at top	10 sec.
Pulse-Up	2	10–12	hold 3 at top	10 sec.
Dumbell Fly	2	10–12	2 down, 3 up	1 min.

DAY TWO (PULL)

EXERCISE	SETS	REPS	REP SPEED (SEC)	REST INTERVAL
Barbell Squat	2	10–12	2 down, explode up	1 min.
Leg Curl	2	10–12	2 down, 3 up	1 min.
Biceps Curl	2	10–12	2 down, 3 up	1 min.
Bent-Over Row 2	2	10–12	2 down, 3 up	2 min.
Lateral Pulldown	2	10–12	2 down, 3 up	1 min.
Calf Raise	2	10–12	2 down, 3 up	1 min.
Reverse Crunch	2	10–12	2 down, 2 up	1 min.
Twisting Oblique Crunch	2	10–12	2 down, 2 up	1 min.

POSITIONS OF STRENGTH ▶

After a dizzying 54 pages of workouts, how can there be more? The next 13 exercises are specifically targeted to sexual positions mentioned in this book and are the most effective workout for the position they're paired with. For example, the missionary position works best if you support your weight over your partner's body, leaving some space in between. What bears the bulk of that effort? Your shoulders— and the best exercise to strengthen them is the lateral raise.

The positions we chose range from everyday basic to spice-it-up complex. We picked perennial favorites (missionary, woman on top) as well as ones we think you'll like even if you don't try them more than once (the Honeybee, the Pretzel).

You can incorporate each exercise into the workouts described earlier in this chapter by prioritizing one or two each day at the beginning of your workout. Or, if you're not up for the full exercise program for whatever reason, pick the exercise that supports your favorite position and do that one only. That's an ideal strategy for when you don't have a lot of time to work out or you're on the road or under the weather. Even if you can't get a full workout in, your sex life won't suffer.

Man on Top *(page 58)*

Why she likes it: *Deep penetration, ease of kissing, body-to-body closeness. The so-called missionary position hardly indicates a lack of creativity. Surveys show it's a perennial favorite of men as well as women. In this position, you also can press your pubic bone against her clitoris as you rock and thrust, giving her extreme pleasure.*

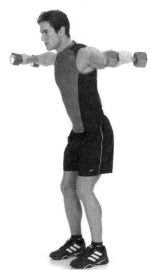

MUSCLES TO WORK: Shoulders. They keep your torso upright and keep your full weight off her body. Also, your naked chest and abs give her extra visual pleasure.

BEST WORKOUT: Standing Lateral Raises. Stand holding a pair of dumbbells at your sides with an overhand grip, your elbows slightly bent. Bend slightly forward at the hips, keeping your lower back in its naturally arched position. Raise your arms up and out to the sides until they're parallel with the floor, keeping the same bend in your elbows. Pause, then slowly return to the starting position. Try for three sets of eight repetitions each.

Woman on Top *(page 65)*

Why she likes it: She controls the pace and movements.

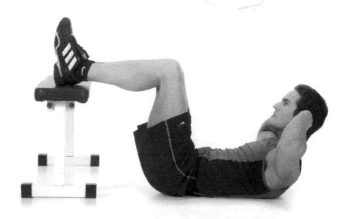

MUSCLES TO WORK: Abdominals. They provide good thrusting control and force—important when you're in the passive position, without the leverage you have on top.

BEST WORKOUT: Crunches. Lie on your back, with your knees bent at 90 degrees or resting on a bench. Hold your hands behind your ears. Use your abs to curl your torso upward 4 to 6 inches, keeping your lower back firmly pressed to the floor. Pause, then slowly lower. Try to start with three sets of 10 crunches. As your endurance increases, increase it to five sets of 20.

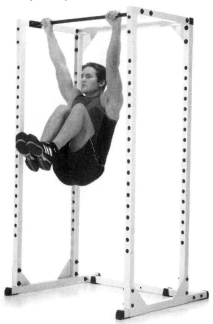

Woman on Top, Back to Front *(page 68)*

Why she likes it: There's deep penetration, she controls the pace, and she can stimulate her clitoris manually. In this classic Eastern position, you lie on your back as the woman straddles your penis, her bottom toward your face.

MUSCLES TO WORK: Hips, abdominals, and thighs. You'll need strength in these areas to rock forward and back and to angle your hips for optimal penetration.

BEST WORKOUT: Hanging Leg Raises. Using a chinup bar and an overhand grip, hang with your arms straight and shoulder-width apart. Use your abdominal muscles to raise your legs until they're a bit higher than your hips. Hold it for 2 seconds, then return to the starting position. Try for three sets of eight repetitions.

Tabletop Sex (*page 89*)

Why she likes it: Spontaneous passion, deep penetration.

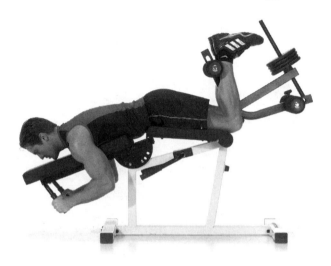

MUSCLES TO WORK: Hamstrings. These muscles have to be strong to have sex while standing, especially when you're bent over and thrusting forward.

BEST WORKOUT: Leg Curls. Lie facedown on a leg-curl machine. With your hips flat against the bench and your abdominal muscles tight, curl your legs behind you until your feet are about perpendicular to the bench. Pause, then lower your legs slowly to the starting position, stopping just before your knees are straight. Try for three sets of eight repetitions.

Sitting (page 82)

Why she likes it: Sex while sitting offers the best of all possible worlds. You can penetrate as deeply as you can in lying positions, with a bonus: The woman gets the opportunity to set the pace, moving as quickly or slowly as she likes.

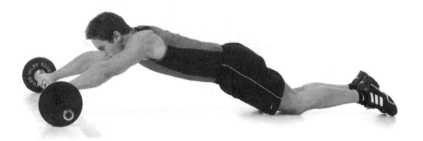

MUSCLES TO WORK: Back and abdominals. Strength in these areas makes it easier to hold yourself and your partner upright without fatigue.

BEST WORKOUT: Wheel of Torture. Kneel on the floor as though doing a modified pushup, with your hands resting on a barbell. Glide forward as you roll the bar in front of you, flexing your shoulders and extending your spine. Keep going until your hips are in line with your torso. Then slide backward until you're back in the kneeling position. Try for three sets of eight repetitions.

Standing, from the Back (page 86)

Why she likes it: Very deep, fast penetration.

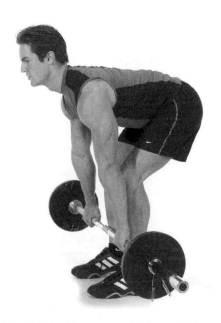

MUSCLES TO WORK: Forearms, back, and biceps. You need to hold your partner firmly to keep from thrusting her into a nosedive.

BEST WORKOUT: Wide-Stance Romanian Deadlift. Stand with your legs hip-width apart and your knees slightly bent. Grab a barbell with an overhand grip and your hands just beyond shoulder-width apart. Hold the bar at arm's length at mid-thigh level with your shoulders back and chest out. Keeping your back flat and your knees slightly bent, bend forward at the hips, keeping the bar close to your thighs. Lower the bar toward the floor, going as far as you comfortably can. Slowly return to the starting position, keeping your back straight throughout the exercise. Try for three sets of eight repetitions.

Skin the Cat *(page 97)*

Why she likes it: The giddy headrush.

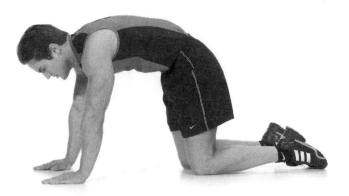

MUSCLES TO WORK: Deep abdominals. When you're on your knees, and your partner straddles you in an upside-down position, you need strong abdominals to hold yourself upright and to move back and forth.

BEST WORKOUT: Kneeling Vacuum. Get down on your hands and knees, keeping your back flat. Take a deep breath, allowing your belly to push out. Then forcibly exhale and round your back as you lift your navel up toward your spine, contracting your pelvic muscles. When you can no longer exhale, keep your back rounded. Hold the contraction for anywhere from 10 to 60 seconds, breathing regularly the whole time. Rest for a minute, then repeat up to 10 times.

The Honeybee (page 99)

Why she likes it: Intense G-spot stimulation with every thrust. This position allows maximum penetration and visual stimulation.

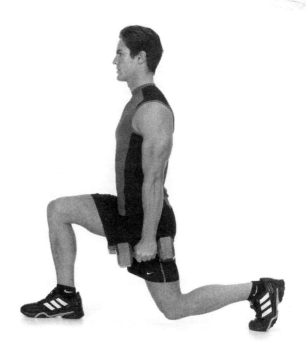

MUSCLES TO WORK: Legs, hips, and butt

BEST WORKOUT: Dumbbell Lunge. Grab a dumbbell in each hand, your palms facing your body, and stand with your feet hip-width apart. Keeping your back straight, take a long step forward with your right leg. Bend your leg until your right thigh is parallel with the floor. Your left leg should be extended, with your knee slightly bent and almost touching the floor. Keep your right foot stationary as you straighten your right leg. Switch legs and repeat on the other side.

Standing (page 86)

Why she likes it: Full body-to-body contact, the feel of your hands on her butt.

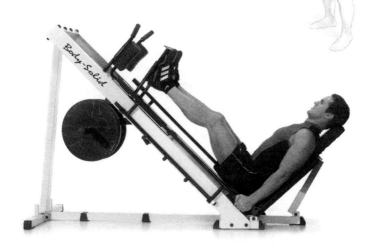

MUSCLES TO WORK: Calves, hamstrings, and butt. They work together to provide the strength needed to hold your partner off the floor.

BEST WORKOUT: Leg Presses, which work all three muscle groups together. Sit on a leg-press machine with your back against the pad and your feet shoulder-width apart on the foot plate. Adjust the seat so your knees are bent slightly more than 90 degrees. Push the weight until your knees are almost locked, then slowly return to the starting position. Try for three sets of eight repetitions.

Rear Entry (page 71)

Why she likes it: Rear-entry (or doggy-style) positions allow for very deep penetration and for manual stimulation of her clitoris by either of you.

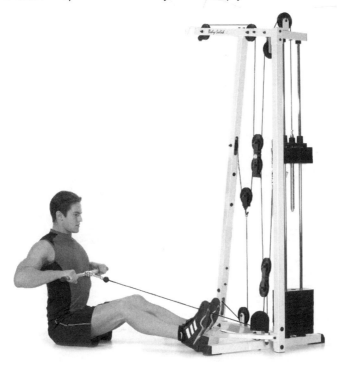

MUSCLES TO WORK: Back. You need a lot of back strength to hold your partner in position–and to hold yourself upright while thrusting forward.

BEST WORKOUT: Cable Seated Row. Sit on the floor, knees bent, and grip the cable handle. Pull the handle straight back until it almost touches your waist; at the same time, pull your shoulders back and push your chest forward. Hold for a moment, then extend your arms as you return to the starting position; your shoulders and lower back should flex forward slightly. Try for three sets of eight repetitions.

Side by Side (page 78)

Why she likes it: There's deep penetration in the spooning variation of the side-by-side position, it's easy for you (or her) to touch her clitoris, and it involves little vigorous thrusting—good when you're both tired.

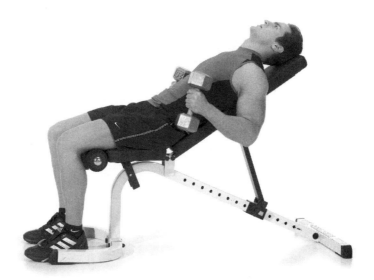

MUSCLES TO WORK: Arms. The penis tends to slip from the vagina with some frequency in this position. You need strong arms to grasp her pelvis and hold her tight.

BEST WORKOUT: Incline Hammer Curl. Sit back on an incline bench with about a 45-degree angle. Hold a dumbbell in each hand, with your arms hanging at your sides. With your palms facing inward and your upper arms still, curl the dumbbells straight up, keeping your wrists locked. You can work both arms simultaneously or, if that's too difficult, alternate arms. Try for two or three sets of eight repetitions each.

Scissors *(page 103)*

Why she likes it: Her clitoris will get extra stimulation as it rubs against your inner thigh during thrusting in this crisscross position.

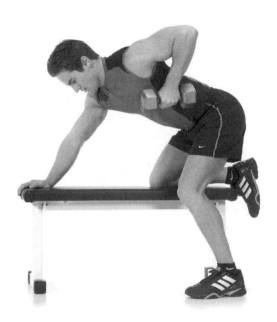

MUSCLES TO WORK: Latissimus dorsi (back muscles). A strong back makes it easier to hold her close when you're in a sitting position.

BEST WORKOUT: One-Arm Dumbbell Row. Holding a dumbbell in your left hand, rest your right knee and right hand on a bench. Keep your back flat as you let the dumbbell hang down to your side so your arm lines up just in front of your shoulder. With your left foot firmly on the floor, knee slightly bent, pull the dumbbell up and in toward your torso, raising it as high as it will go. Try for three sets of eight repetitions, then switch positions and work the other arm.

The Pretzel *(page 111)*

Why she likes it: Access to her clitoris in a comfortable reclining position.

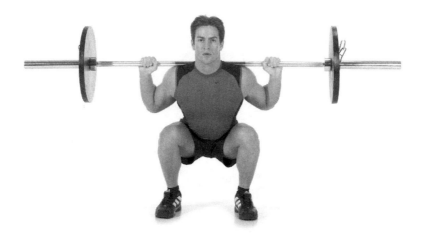

MUSCLES TO WORK: Butt. You have to have strong glutes to hold this position.

BEST WORKOUT: Barbell squats. Place a barbell at shoulder level on a squat rack. Grip the bar with your hands slightly more than shoulder-width apart, palms facing front. Step under the bar so that it's evenly positioned across your upper back and shoulders, not your neck. Stand up straight, with your feet hip-width apart and your knees slightly bent. Don't drop your head; keep it in line with your torso. Keeping your feet flat and torso straight, bend your knees slightly and squat down, as though sitting in a chair behind you. Don't allow your knees to extend past your toes. Continue moving downward until your thighs are parallel to the floor. Then slowly rise to a standing position. Try for three sets of eight repetitions.

CHAPTER 9

YOUR BEATING HEART: THE CARDIOVASCULAR KEY TO GOOD SEX

ATHLETES IN FULL-CONTACT SPORTS CAN COUNT ON TRAINERS TO PUMP THEM FULL OF OXYGEN OR MAS-SAGE THEIR MUSCLES WHEN THEY'RE ON THE BRINK OF COLLAPSE. Sad to say, you can't get the same kind of help if your body suddenly gives out in the bedroom. If you like the idea of having sex all night, get used to the idea that your successes or failures are entirely up to you.

"There is nothing more embarrassing than panting and gasping when performing even the simplest moves," a 24-year-old computer support specialist in Montclair, New Jersey, told us. *"I almost always get tired and have to rest,"* added a 52-year-old technical writer.

Here's a simple fact about the human male: He needs air. If you can't breathe, you can't make love, at least not very well. Guys who are out of shape may notice that they can't have sex and talk at the same time. They have trouble when they try to talk *and* have sex *and* change positions a few times.

There are all sorts of solutions to the kinds of sexual problems that pain men most, such as coming too quickly or not getting hard (or hard enough) when they want to. These are critical issues that deserve all the attention they get. But the foundation, the *heart* of good sex always comes down to air. Vigorous sex requires endurance no less than an erection. If your cardiovascular system can't cut it, neither will you.

More is involved than just kissing and breathing at the same time. Your entire body pays the price if your heart and lungs don't work at peak capacity.

▶ A lot of muscles come into play when you have sex. Each of them requires an abundant flow of oxygen. Limit the amount of air that comes in—and the amount of carbon dioxide that's carted out—and your strength will plummet. You'll tire easily. You'll be more likely to get debilitating, sex-stopping cramps.

▶ Blood flows to the most active muscles when you're having sex. At the same time, it continues to circulate to other body systems. If your heart isn't pounding efficiently, circulation can be significantly compromised. No, you won't die (probably), but there may be a drop in the system-wide distribution of nutrients, hormones, or other key chemicals that you need for full energy and arousal.

▶ The landmark Massachusetts Male Aging Study, which tracked more than 600 middle-age and older men for more than 10 years, found that those who weren't active had twice the risk of impotence compared with those who took a brisk, 2-mile walk daily. Another study, this one at the New England Research Institute in Watertown, Massachusetts, reported that 31 percent of sedentary men developed impotence, compared with only 9 percent who whipped their cardiovascular systems into shape.

No matter how much you lift weights, no matter how many games of golf you play, no matter how often you sort through all the clothes that you've heaped on the now-invisible exercise bike, you have to add cardiovascular workouts into your life. You'll notice that we didn't say that you might want to think about it. You *have* to do it—to save your sex life as well as your life.

Stamina originates with a strong heart. The best way to strengthen the heart is with aerobic workouts: jogging, fast walking,

CAN A MAN FAKE AN ORGASM?

Of course. Men can fake anything. Unlike a woman's orgasm, however, men leave a little something behind. Even if your partner doesn't feel the spurt of semen—and many women don't—she's bound to notice something's amiss.

A better question to ask yourself is why you'd even want to fake an orgasm. It's true that women (and men) sometimes fake orgasms to make their partners feel better or simply to end a sexual session for whatever reason. But this kind of deception, however well intentioned, isn't as harmless as it appears. Once you start faking anything, and once you get caught (as you will eventually), your partner will start wondering what else you lie about. Maybe, her thinking might go, you're not really attracted to her. Maybe you just pretend to like her in bed. Maybe you just pretend to like her, *period.*

Faking an orgasm might be a time-honored way to let your partner (and yourself) off the hook, but the possible repercussions aren't worth it. Besides, you want to have the kind of relationship that fosters sexual openness, not deceit. Who cares if you (or your partner) don't come on occasion? It's normal. Why lie about it?

swimming, cycling, and so on. Any time you kick your heart rate up a few notches and keep it there for half an hour or so, your heart muscle gets stronger, and your resting heart rate declines. The lungs get more efficient. Blood pressure goes down. Circulation goes up. And on and on.

"I started running a few years ago, and my endurance went way up. Believe it or not, I have better erections now than I did when I was 30 because I don't party any more, and I work out regularly," a 45-year-old contractor in Tucson told us.

"I meet a lot more women than I used to, probably because my body image and confidence is a lot higher since I started aerobic training," says a 23-year-old student in Madison, Wisconsin.

What else can you get from regular cardiovascular training? Take a look.

▶ **An increase in sex drive.** A study of more than 8,000 people ages 18 to 45 found that 40 percent had increases in sexual arousal after starting a regular exercise program. One-third of them reported that they had sex more often.

▶ **Better orgasms.** Researchers at the University of California report that sedentary middle-age men who started exercising for 1 hour three times weekly had better orgasms, better erections, and higher overall sexual satisfaction.

▶ **More testosterone.** Aerobic workouts stimulate the body's production of testosterone, the hormone that stimulates libido and promotes erections.

▶ **Less fat.** Sure, you can lose weight (or at least fat) by lifting weights, but it's a slow way to do it. Cardiovascular training puts you on the fast track. Men who walk at a leisurely, 4-mile-an-hour pace for 30 minutes will burn about 240 calories, 40 percent of which come from fat. Men who exercise more vigorously can count on burning lard at up to *eight times* the normal rate.

▶ **Less death.** Well, that's a bit of a stretch, but cardiovascular conditioning dramatically reduces the risk of heart attack, the leading cause of death in American men and women. It also cuts the risk of diabetes and colon cancer as well as high blood pressure.

▶ **A better mood.** The brain churns out endorphins, opiate-like brain chemicals that make you feel calm and self-assured, when you kick-start your cardiovascular system. The same chemicals that account for the runner's high can cut your risk of depression and anxiety while boosting levels of confidence and self-esteem.

WHY AEROBICS?

The terms *aerobics* and *aerobic exercise* are often used interchangeably, but they aren't quite the same thing. Aerobics generally refers to aerobic dance—leotards, mirrored walls, and nerve-grating, upbeat music. Aerobic exercise, by contrast, means any exercise that gets your heart pumping faster than usual—and keeps it at that rate for an extended period.

Strictly speaking, any activity performed faster than sitting in a chair is aerobic. But to produce any real benefit, there has to be substantial physical effort involved—which is why you won't see billiard players on the Olympic medal stand any time in the near future. True aerobic exercise, the kinds of workouts that tax your heart and lungs as well as your muscles, requires that you push yourself to roughly 60 to 90 percent of your maximum ability. More simply, you get an aerobic workout—also known as cardiovascular exercise—when you significantly raise your heartbeat for at least 30 minutes at a stretch.

Not so long ago, nearly everyone earned their daily crust through hard, physical labor. Aerobic workouts were pretty much a given. Lately, though, we've all gotten more sedentary. If you spend your days doing nothing more physically taxing than fingering computer keys, and your nightly activity is jamming buttons on the remote control, you can bet that your heart and lungs aren't doing what they should—and your sex life, including your ability to even *want* a sex life, is probably paying the price.

Scientists first started examining the link between physical activity and the heart in the 1960s. Harvard and Stanford scientists discovered that longshoremen who were promoted to management positions developed heart disease at a much higher rate than the guys who stayed on the dock. They surmised that hard physical activity had significant cardio-protecting effects—and decades of subsequent research proved them right.

Men in some African tribes run while maintaining erections. They believe that it increases sexual stamina.

For a long time, researchers were pretty sure that cardiovascular workouts had a significant health edge over non-aerobic types of exercise, such as weight lifting or short sprints. There's no question that you really have to push the heart and lungs to achieve true cardiovascular fitness. For cardiovascular *health,* however, you don't have to sweat anywhere near as hard as people once thought. Almost any kind of exercise, even leisurely walking, can extend your life and reduce the risk of diabetes, high blood pressure, and other diseases. But the basic premise of cardiovascular training is still true: Pushing your heart and lungs past their usual comfort zones can extend your life *and* improve your sex life.

When you engage in any kind of exercise—anything from mowing the grass to making love—muscle cells are suddenly stressed. Roused from their lassitude, they demand a quick infusion of blood and oxygen. The heart responds by pumping harder and faster in order to route more blood through the lungs for oxygenation. As long as the exercise continues, the muscles continuously demand more blood, and the heart and lungs keep working at an accelerated rate.

The heart, keep in mind, is a muscle, one that gets stronger the harder you work it. As the heart gets more buffed, it starts doing the same amount of work with less effort. That's why men who work out tend to have lower resting heart rates than those who are sedentary.

The blood vessels get stronger and more elastic when you start cardiovascular training. Circulation improves throughout the body, including in the tiny blood vessels that carry blood through the penis and make erections possible. Men who start almost any kind of cardiovascular training have better bloodflow with lower blood pressure. They're less likely to develop the kinds of vascular disease that can put their sex lives out of commission. And they're more likely to have the extra energy and libido that can push their erotic pleasures to another level.

THE AEROBIC BOTTOM LINE

The President's Council on Fitness has identified four essential components—the ABCDs—of cardiovascular fitness.

▶ Amount. For optimal fitness, strive for a workout intensity that pushes your heart rate to 65 to 85 percent of its maximum capacity. We'll talk more about this in just a bit. In the meantime, don't let the numbers throw you. You can ballpark it by exercising with an intensity somewhere between fairly light and fairly hard. Even if you don't quite hit the target range, you'll get nearly all of the benefits, minus a percentage point or two.

▶ **Best type.** This one's easy. The best aerobic workout is one that you'll actually do. Doesn't matter if it's jumping rope, swimming laps, or running hard a few steps ahead of the IRS. If you do it regularly, you'll get fit.

▶ **Consistency.** Good intentions don't count. For optimal sexual (and physical and emotional) health, you need to set aside time 3 to 5 days a week. Don't expect to get the same benefits if you blow off your workouts for 3 weeks, then pound yourself into a frenzy a few days in a row. Consistency is everything—and that goes for downtime as well. When you're starting out, plan on resting for a day or two between workouts. Time off is especially important if you're running or doing other high-impact activities.

▶ **Duration.** Plan on exercising for 30 to 60 minutes each time. That's a huge range, of course, but it doesn't seem to matter all that much exactly where in the range you fall. Recent studies show that men can get nearly the same health benefits from a 30-minute workout as they can from a full hour.

Since the core of any aerobic workout requires boosting the heart rate above its usual level, it's worth taking a little time to explain exactly what this means—and how to customize your workouts to shove your heart into the optimal zone.

Optimal, incidentally, doesn't mean "the most you can do before you die." Don't launch into cardiovascular training with the idea that your heart needs to be beating so hard that it bulges from your chest; that sweat should be spouting from every pore; and that your head will be pounding as though it's about to explode, either shortly before or after you pass out.

With the possible exception of Richard Simmons videos, aerobic workouts shouldn't be painful. You simply need to elevate your heartbeat until it reaches what is known as your target heart rate. This isn't defined by the outer limits of your heart's endurance. Rather, it represents your aerobic range—roughly 60 to 90 percent of the maximum rate your heart is capable of. (Although the President's Council recommends 65 to 85 percent, 60 to 90 percent is more realistic.)

A huge amount of research has shown that this is the ideal exercise range. For example, researchers at the University of California in San Diego looked at 78 healthy but sedentary men. Some were assigned to a "couch group" to act as controls. The others enrolled in a 9-month program of aerobic exercise in which the intensity of the workouts—walking at a moderate pace for 60 minutes 4 days a week—pushed their hearts into the aerobic range.

Men in the exercise group not only reported having more sex than those who were sedentary, they also enjoyed it more. And the more they exercised, the better the sex got.

Every man has a different target heart rate. The easiest way to identify your personal range is to subtract your age from 220 and multiply that by 0.6 to get the lower end of the range, then again by 0.9 to get the upper figure.

If you're 40, for example, you'd first subtract your age from 220 (answer: 180). Multiply that by 0.6 to get 108. That's the lower end of your aerobic range. Now, start again. Multiply 180 by 0.9 to get 162. That's the upper end of your range. Now you know what you're shooting for.

Just to make things a little more complicated, studies have shown that people who've been sedentary for a lot of years can improve their aerobic fitness by starting with a target heart rate as low as 40 percent of max. This time, subtract your age from 220 and multiply that number by 0.4. Once you're in better shape, you can kick it up into the 60 to 90 percent range.

Checking your pulse isn't the only way to rate the intensity of aerobic exercise. Here are some other options.

▶ A heart-rate monitor. They're easy to use, inexpensive if you don't get all the bells and whistles, and available at just about any sporting goods store.

▶ The talk test. This is one of the best techniques because there are no equations, no stopping to check your pulse, and almost no thought. All you have to do is ask yourself if you have enough wind during exercise to talk at the same time. As you might expect, scientists have given this technique its own gaudy name: the Talk Test Method (TTM). It can be quite

FEELING THE BEAT

Forget what you see on *ER:* Taking an accurate pulse isn't always easy, especially during exercise, when your chest is heaving, and you're sucking every bit of air you can muster. Here's the easiest way to do it.

▶ Locate the carotid artery, the big pipe in your neck that runs alongside the windpipe and Adam's apple. If you look closely, you'll see it pulsing with each beat.

▶ Put your finger on the artery so you can feel the pulse. Count the beats for 10 seconds, then multiply that number by six. That's your heart rate per minute. Pressing too hard on the artery will skew the count. Also, don't use your thumb; it has its own pulse, which can complicate things.

▶ Take the reading within 10 seconds of pausing during exercise. If you wait longer than that, your heart rate will drop quickly. You may think you're not exercising hard enough, when in fact you may have reached your target heart range or even gone beyond it. Pushing yourself beyond that range is neither necessary nor safe.

useful in determining your aerobic comfort zone, particularly when you're just starting out. If you're able to talk during your workout without a great deal of strain, you're most likely in your comfort zone.

▶ Borg Rating of Perceived Exertion. It's a useful measure of exercise intensity because it basically rates how you feel. On a scale of 10, the average man engaged in aerobic exercise should rate his physical and mental fatigue somewhere between 4 and 6. The scale looks something like this:

0–1: No exertion. You're either watching TV, sleeping, or dead. Breathing is so slight, it's barely noticeable.

2–3: Minimal exertion. For example, working on the computer (non-porn sites only) or easy walking. Breathing is normal, and conversation is easy.

4–5: Moderate exertion. Jogging or fast walking, for example. Breathing is getting harder.

6–7: Very strong exertion. You might be running, cycling, or swimming. Breathing is heavy.

8–9: Close to maximum exertion. Sprinting will get you there. You're struggling to breathe.

10: Maximum exertion. This would be an all-out sprint. You're absolutely at your limit.

It's worth mentioning that all of these techniques and numbers apply only to men in good health. If you're 40 years or older or have risk factors for heart disease (such as smoking or high cholesterol), talk to your doctor before starting any kind of exercise plan. You might be advised to take it far slower than the guidelines advise, at least until you get into better shape.

DESIGN YOUR WORKOUT

As we mentioned earlier, you have to pick a cardiovascular workout that you really and truly enjoy. Otherwise, you'll find it hard to get out of bed in the morning, much less out the door. Of course, it's possible that you don't even *need* to add exercise to your life. If you live in a cozy home in rural Vermont, for example, and you spend your days cutting, hauling, and stacking firewood to fend off the brutal cold, you're probably already getting all the aerobic exercise that you need. The same if you live in a 20th-floor walk-up in New York City, and you go up and down the stairs a dozen times a day.

Most of us, though, need some kind of "artificial" exercise. What's it to be? Walking? Jogging? Running? Swimming? Prizefighting? Sure, they're all good. So are a million other things. Walking fast to the supermarket instead of driving. Loping along behind the lawnmower. It doesn't matter what you do, as long as it kicks your heart into the target range and keeps it there for at least 30 minutes. Your heart doesn't know the difference between "real" exercise and simply moving quickly.

If you've practiced exercise avoidance most of your life, you'll obviously want to start slowly. More than a few guys haul themselves off the couch, go out and spend $1,000 on a new bike, then irritate the heck out of their friends when they call from the next county needing a ride home. Moving too quickly into exercise will only cause fatigue, sore muscles, and mental and physical burnout.

So where do you start? Just in case you're wondering, sex probably won't do it. Yes, it provides a vigorous workout. But unless you can keep it up for 30 minutes three or four times a week, stopping periodically to take your pulse to ensure you're in the target range, you'd better not count on it. Here are some more practical options.

DO IT WITH CLASS. Just about every health club offers a range of cardiovascular workout classes. Traditional aerobics classes were dominated by women, and many still are—but don't assume that they're lightweight. Just about any class will give you a killer workout. If the so-called aerobic dance workouts aren't for you, you have other options: Spinning, aero-boxing (or plain boxing), and jump-roping, to name a few. They're often geared to men, although plenty of women take them, too.

GO UP A LEVEL. How many times have you walked right past the stairs at your apartment complex or office? You're ignoring one of the best aerobic workouts you can get. Climbing stairs—and coming back down—puts tremendous strain on the quadriceps, hamstring, butt, hip, and calf muscles. It puts an equally hard strain on the heart and lungs. In fact, researchers say that the exertion of sex is the equivalent of climbing stairs, so you can think of it as a kind of training.

Best of all, stairclimbing is free. No membership fees, no fancy clothes, and no waiting in line when linebacker-size dudes form packs around the dumbbell rack.

RIDE YOURSELF RAGGED. Cycling is a great workout for the legs, lungs, and heart. More and more men are doing it, either on the road or in Spinning classes, because it's a lot easier on the knees and back than running. It's also more fun than a lot of other aerobic workouts, which is probably why men who take up a cycling program tend to stick with it.

GET YOUR OARS WET. If you're lucky enough to live in an area with a lake or river, rowing, also known as sculling, is probably the best cardiovascular workout you can get. A NASA study found that rowing consistently burns 15 to 20 percent more calories than cycling—and you don't have to worry about flat tires.

The rowing machines at gyms are good substitutes, especially those with sliding seats. They'll quickly build your back, arms, butt, and legs and provide a tough workout for your heart and lungs as well.

GIVE RUNNING ANOTHER CHANCE. It's true that millions of men have tried running, and an almost equal number hate it. The reason for running's spotty reputation is that too many men go all out. They force themselves to run longer, faster, and harder and eventually collapse with blasted knees—or at least get sick of the chronically sore ankles, shins, and feet that seem almost inevitable.

But if you run smart—that is, staying below the threshold of fatigue and soreness—running is a superb workout. Even running at a sedate, 12-minute-mile pace will burn roughly 10 calories a minute. Then there's the simplicity factor. You don't have to learn a lot about technique. Just put one foot in front of the other.

Running does put a lot of stress on your body. Each time your foot hits the ground, it strikes with a force equal to three to four times your body weight. You have to be sensible—by running on grass, for example; replacing your shoes every 3 to 6 months; and warming up before runs and cooling down after.

GET IN THE SWIM. Swimming is easier on the back, ligaments, and joints than running. It burns a tremendous amount of calories. It requires you to use just about all of your major muscle groups, while stimulating the cardiovascular system at an impressive level. Water gives 12 times the resistance of air, which is why a 180-pound guy can burn 630 calories an hour doing a slow crawl—about the same as running for an hour on hilly terrain.

The water isn't our natural environment, of course, and swimming takes some practice to achieve a reasonable level of expertise. Definitely consider getting qualified instruction if you aren't a natural. Invest in good goggles to minimize the chlorine sting. And give some thought to the suit you'll be comfortable in. A standard-issue racing suit offers virtually no drag in the water, but it will reveal parts of your anatomy that only your intimates are familiar with. The standard beach britches work fine for most guys.

TAKE A WALK. It's never been accorded much respect by the more macho exercise elements, but look at the facts. Men who walk at a moderate pace get the same cardiovascular benefits as those who jog. Then there's the injury factor: It doesn't happen when you walk. If you can get up from the couch, you can walk. No trainers or specialized gear needed.

Walking does take time, though, a scarce commodity in today's world. To get the best results, you'll probably want to walk for about 45 minutes most days of the week. Why not make it fun? Take your dog. Use the time to catch up with your friends. Meet women at the park. You're going to be out there anyway; you might as well enjoy it.

▼

A modest pucker utilizes two facial muscles, but a full-fledged, passionate kiss employs 34. Result: A 1-minute kiss burns roughly 26 calories.

▲

TRY WALKING-PLUS. True, walking is a superb way to ease into an aerobic workout program. It's easy to do; it's easy on the joints; it's easy to enjoy. On the other hand, it doesn't exactly get your adrenaline pumping. Some men enjoy the mental peace they get from walking. Others, within a few weeks, find that they're bored out of their minds.

Part of the problem is that men tend to approach walking as a pleasant stroll. That's good for enjoyment, and it's okay for your heart. Okay, but not great. The only way to transform a stroll into a heart-pounding, 30- to 45-minute workout is to pump it up.

▶ Walk slowly for 5 to 10 minutes to warm up.

▶ Pick up your pace to 4 to 5 miles an hour. You should be swinging your arms, not letting them dangle at your sides. After a few minutes, you should be breathing harder, and your heart rate will be picking up.

▶ Choose a route that includes some hills. Walking at an angle stresses the muscles in different ways and increases the rush of blood through the heart and lungs.

▶ Pick up the pace some more. Again, you want to be breathing hard, but not so hard that you're sucking air. Remember the rule we mentioned earlier: Your breathing should be labored, yet you should have sufficient reserves to talk at the same time.

▶ Kick into a gentle jog, somewhere between fast walking and running. After a few minutes of that, increase your pace to a full jog. That's where you're going to stay for the duration of your outing. You don't want to break into a run, because it's hard on the joints. A steady jog will take you along at a speed that's two to three times faster than when you started.

▶ Slow down for the last few minutes of your route. Slow from a jog to fast walking, and then to a leisurely stroll. This cooldown time gives your heart and lungs a chance to recover, and it flushes lactic acid from your leg muscles.

Men who stick to a walking-plus program usually find that their resting heart rates have significantly slowed within a few weeks. The needle on the scale won't swing quite as far to the right. You'll have toned your body as well as your lungs. And you'll probably find that you have more strength and endurance in the bedroom because your overall energy has spiked upward. Ultimately, that's what this is all about.

INTERVAL TRAINING

Aerobic training is terrific for cardiovascular health, but it's not so great at building strength or burning fat. Sure, you can have great sex if you're overweight, and you hardly need the muscles of a pro wrestler to play with most positions. But a man who's lean is generally more attractive to women—and a man who *feels* lean and confident will definitely get more attention. The trick is to add fuel to your usual aerobic workouts with a technique known as interval training—slipping high-intensity exercises into your normal routine.

The idea is simple enough. Whatever level of exercise you're accustomed to eventually becomes routine; progress slows or stops. Trainers call this phase a plateau, and it's frustrating because all of your hard work doesn't seem to be adding up to much. The only way to break through the plateau is to give your body challenges it hasn't had before.

With interval training, you alternate bouts of vigorous, *anaerobic* exercise with your usual aerobic sessions. Here's an example. Suppose you've been running for a few months—nothing crazy, but solid and consistent. It's become as easy as breathing. Your muscles aren't challenged, your lungs aren't challenged, and your mind definitely isn't challenged. So you throw a little extra something into the mix—say, periodic sprints that stress the muscles in a way that routine running doesn't. The added stress tears down muscle fibers. They're forced to rebuild themselves, which translates into an increase in strength and size.

Another benefit of interval training is that it promotes faster weight loss. Aerobic workouts do burn fat, but only after you've already burned your available supply of carbohydrates—and the benefits stop when the exercise does. When you throw an anaerobic workout into the mix, you burn fat right away and keep burning it even after exercise is over. At the same time, the stressed muscles continue the rebuilding process even when you're lounging on the couch.

Here are the basics.

▶ Several times a week, intersperse your regular workout—jogging, cycling, whatever—with high-intensity, strength-building exertion.

▶ The aerobic part of your workout should be done at an intensity of 50 to 70 percent of your target heart rate. The anaerobic phase should kick you into the 80 to 90 percent range. (Check with your doctor before pushing your exercise intensity to these maximum levels.)

▶ The anaerobic phase of your workouts should last 2 to 10 minutes. Continue interspersing bursts of high-intensity exercise. For example, walk or jog at your usual steady pace for 2 minutes. Then walk or run hard for 2 minutes. Then switch back to the slower pace. Repeat each interval eight times.

▶ Allow yourself plenty of rest during interval training. If you're getting winded or sore, take a break for a few minutes, then resume your exercise.

▶ Always start with a warmup. For example, start out by walking for 5 to 10 minutes, keeping your heart rate at about 50 to 60 percent of its target range. Then increase the intensity to your usual level and from there, kick in with the intervals.

THE COOLDOWN PHASE

Trainers always advise men to end aerobic workouts with a cooldown period, and men just as often ignore them. Yes, it takes a couple of minutes that you'd probably rather use for something else, and yes, it's a little on the boring side. Do it anyway. Stopping suddenly after hard exercise puts unnecessary strain on the heart. You can pass out if your blood pressure

UNSEXY SMOKING

It wasn't that long ago that the U.S. government supplied soldiers with free packs of Lucky Strikes, and lab-coated physicians appeared on television commercials to extol the health benefits of charcoal-filtered Larks. For a long time, cigarettes were considered the pinnacle of class and sophistication.

We know today, of course, that smoking is a dangerous habit, one that kills an estimated 400,000 Americans a year. We won't hammer you with the litany of risks; you know them all by heart. Suffice it to say that smoking is a common cause of impotence. Chemicals in the smoke cause blood vessels to clamp down. Less blood means you won't get as hard as you should, if you even get hard at all. Smoking even makes the erectile tissue in the penis less sensitive to stimulation.

If you're a smoker and are thinking about trying to quit, well, you have our sympathy. The tobacco habit is even harder to kick than heroin. There are plenty of stop-smoking approaches that can make it a little easier. Patches, for example, suffuse your body with nicotine while you try to beat the habit. Nicotine gum is another option. There are also drugs such as Zyban (bupropion) that can minimize cravings.

Once you quit, you have about a 3-day window of real suffering. That's about how long it takes to clear your body of the physical addiction to nicotine. After that, the craving is mainly psychological. Your body is no longer hooked, but all of your habits—having a smoke with your morning coffee, for example—will do everything in their power to drag you back in. This psychological craving is the toughest to beat.

People who say it's easy to quit have obviously never smoked. It is hard—quite possibly the hardest thing you've ever done. Do it anyway. If you fail the first time, as you probably will, keep trying. Don't hesitate to ask your doctor for help. When you quit, you'll have the satisfaction of knowing you'll live longer. You'll have more energy, you'll breathe better, and you'll have a better time in bed. Go for it.

drops too far. And you'll almost certainly have pain later because you didn't take the time to flush out the lactic acid that accumulates during exercise.

At the end of your workout, take about 5 minutes to cool down with slow, easy exercise. Walk slowly after a hard jog—or jog slowly after a hard run. Cycle at a breathe-easy pace. Do some stretches and breathe deeply. All you're trying to do at this point is avoid shocking your system and keep blood from pooling in your legs and feet.

PROGRAMS YOU CAN USE

There are as many effective cardiovascular training programs as there are men to invent them. Since just about any activity, done quickly, puts beneficial stress on the heart and lungs, and since every man enjoys different things, the potential permutations are endless. But we've gone ahead and created a few basic, ready-to-go programs to make it easier: one for beginners, one for intermediate exercisers, and one for the hard-core contingent.

CARDIOVASCULAR TRAINING, PHASE 1

If you're just starting to get in shape, plan on three cardiovascular sessions a week, using a technique known as continuous training. In other words, pick one cardiovascular exercise and do it for the full duration of your workout. You can do anything you want on different days, but make each day consistent. For example, ride a stationary bike, swim, or fast-walk for 30 to 45 minutes at a pop, making sure that your target heart rate clocks in at around 50 to 60 percent of your top capacity for at least 20 minutes of the workout.

Incidentally, don't be surprised if you notice a sudden drop in energy once you launch into your program. This is normal. Within a few weeks, you'll rebound to your previous level, then surpass it.

▶ **MONDAY:** 10-minute warmup; 20 minutes of continuous exercise; 5-minute cooldown.

▶ **TUESDAY:** Take the day off. And quit complaining: It wasn't that bad.

▶ **WEDNESDAY:** 10-minute warmup; 20 minutes of continuous exercise; 5-minute cooldown.

▶ **THURSDAY:** Rest.

▶ **FRIDAY:** 10 minute warmup; 20 minutes of continuous exercise; 5-minute cooldown.

▶ **SATURDAY** and **SUNDAY**: Rest.

CARDIOVASCULAR TRAINING, PHASE 2

Most men who start a cardiovascular training program can expect to lose at least 1 pound a week.

This workout is designed for men who are in pretty good shape. If you've stuck with Phase 1 of the program for a few months or are otherwise active, it's time to push yourself. Here, the workout intensity is higher. You'll want to increase your target heart rate to 60 to 75 percent of your top capacity. You'll also work out more—4 or 5 days a week instead of 3.

You'll also notice that the workout is more varied. On each day of exercise, do something different: running, swimming, biking, climbing stairs, whatever. We've given exercise examples—but they're just that. Feel free to replace them with whatever aerobic activity you like best.

▶ **MONDAY:** 10-minute warmup; 25 minutes of continuous exercise—say, biking—at 70 percent of your maximum heart rate; 10-minute cooldown.

▶ **TUESDAY:** Rest.

▶ **WEDNESDAY:** 10-minute warmup; swim for 35 minutes at 70 percent of your maximum heart rate; 10-minute cooldown.

▶ **THURSDAY:** 10 minute warmup; bike for 45 minutes at 60 percent of your maximum heart rate; 5-minute cooldown.

▶ **FRIDAY:** Rest.

▶ **SATURDAY:** Do a shorter, higher-intensity workout: 10 minute warmup at 50 percent of your maximum heart rate; 20 minutes on the bike at 75 percent; 10-minute cooldown.

▶ **SUNDAY:** Rest. Or repeat Saturday's workout.

CARDIOVASCULAR TRAINING, PHASE 3

Make no mistake: This is a tough workout. Don't try it unless you've been getting regular aerobic exercise for about a year. As with Phase 2, do whatever exercises you like best.

▶ **MONDAY:** 10-minute warmup; 45 minutes of exercise at 75 percent of your maximum heart rate; 10-minute cooldown.

▶ **TUESDAY:** 15-minute warmup at 50 to 60 percent of your maximum heart rate; 50 minutes of exercise at 70 to 75 percent; 5-minute cooldown.

▶ **WEDNESDAY:** 10-minute warmup at 50 to 60 percent; spend the next 20 minutes switching between hard (90 percent of your maximum heart rate) and moderate (50 percent) exercise, alternating every 2 minutes; 10-minute cooldown.

▶ **THURSDAY:** Rest.

▶ **FRIDAY:** 10-minute warmup at 50 to 60 percent of your maximum heart rate; 20 minutes of exercise at 80 percent; 10-minute cooldown.

▶ **SATURDAY:** 10-minute warmup at 50 to 60 percent; 50 minutes of exercise at 70 to 75 percent; throw in 10 minutes of hard biking, swimming, running, or whatever in your routine; 5-minute cooldown.

▶ **SUNDAY:** Rest.

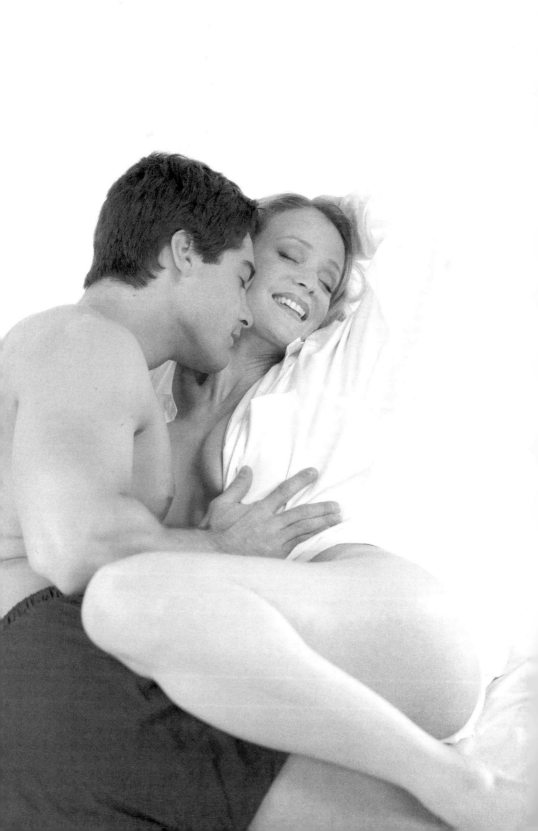

PART 4

FUEL FOR LOVE

CHAPTER 10

THE *BUILT FOR SEX* EATING PLAN

UNLESS YOU'VE BEEN IN A COMA FOR THE PAST 20 YEARS, YOU ALREADY KNOW THAT WHAT YOU EAT IS PROBABLY THE MOST IMPORTANT FACTOR IN HOW YOU LOOK, HOW YOU FEEL, AND, YEP, HOW YOU PERFORM IN BED.

So why is it that so many of us continue to eat the human equivalent of dog food?

Boredom, maybe? Nothing glazes the eyes faster than the words *diet* and *nutrition*. You can't pick up a newspaper or walk through a bookstore without almost getting knocked over by finger-pointing paperbacks with glib advice on what you should eat (and probably aren't), how to lose weight (eventually), and how to cook foods that you don't even want to throw in the compost pile, let alone prepare.

Besides, men today are busier than they've ever been. Who wants to take the time to cram even more guilt-producing information into the brain? Which is why we created the *Built for Sex* Eating Plan. It takes into account your real life, your preferences, and the habits you probably already have. The truth is, all of the nutritional basics that you need to lose weight, look better, and have better sex are just about short enough to fit in a fortune cookie: Cut back on fatty foods, meat, and snacks, and eat more grains, beans, fish, fruits, and vegetables.

Easy, sure—but most of us still don't do it. One survey found that while we're supposed to eat five to nine servings of fruits and vegetables a day, we eat closer to three-and-a-half servings. When you take women out of the mix (they tend to eat more of the good stuff than men do), only about one in five of us eats as many servings of these good foods as we should.

Meanwhile, we're eating a lot more meat and junk food than we need to. Forget for the moment that these kinds of eating habits

LIQUID ASSETS

Doctors have long advised men to drink at least eight glasses of water daily to improve digestive and urinary health as well as to help the body's cells, including those in the penis and testicles, operate at peak efficiency.

But what if you just can't stand water? Try to get used to it; chilling it may help, or adding lemon or lime. If you simply can't stomach the eight tall ones, nature has a few alternatives.

▶ Eat fruit. Apples, grapes, peaches, nectarines—all fresh fruits are mainly water. Eating three to five servings a day will help top off your tank.

▶ Juice it. Buy it fresh and run it through the blender or juicer. Don't filter it: You'll get more fiber, along with all of the vitamins, minerals, and phytochemicals found in whole fruit.

▶ Buy store-bought juice. The best ones are organic: unfiltered, unprocessed, and unsweetened.

vastly increase your risk of diabetes, heart disease, and a variety of cancers. Forget, too, that we're eating ourselves into shapes that resemble the Goodyear blimp. Let's focus instead on what really counts: A lousy diet is literally death to good sex. In too many cases, it's death to *any* sex. This isn't an exaggeration. The kinds of foods that men generally prefer are precisely the ones that can shut down circulation to the place you need it most. We're not talking about heart disease; that comes later. The blood vessels in the penis—the ones that you need to get and sustain an erection—are a heck of a lot smaller than the big pipes in the heart. The foods you eat today can start jamming those arteries long before a cardiologist with a worried look on his face locks you in his office and basically toe-tags you.

Here's the bottom line. The traditional, "I'll worry about it tomorrow" male style of eating is high in saturated fats and trans fats and low in vitamins, minerals, and fiber. It's a perfect prescription for low energy and flagging sexual performance. The *Built for Sex* plan does the opposite. It will give you more energy than you know what to do with. It will improve bloodflow and keep you healthy. It will load your bloodstream with chemical compounds that increase libido as well as your ability to get erections. That's a lot of gain from an eating plan that's almost absurdly simple to follow—and doesn't require you to give up *any* of your favorite foods.

SURVIVAL OF THE FITTEST

You know that fueling your body with nutritious foods is the only way to achieve superior performance. Every professional sports team employs nutritionists. They don't do it for window dressing. They do it because athletes who perform at their physical peaks make a lot of money for the franchise. Those who don't, get traded. Few of us will ever have the power of Jason Giambi or the agility of

Derek Jeter; diet will take you only so far. But every one of us can feel and perform significantly better by incorporating at least some of the principles of athletic nutrition into our daily lives.

"A better diet has given me an increased libido and more energy," a 50-year-old retired engineer told us. Or consider these words from a 24-year-old musician in Manhattan. He didn't give up his fast-lane lifestyle, far from it. But he did start eating better after one of his best friends and fellow musicians barely made it out of rehab alive. *"I can't stress enough how much more energy and stamina I've attained through eating properly,"* he said. *"Before, I didn't always have enough energy to have sex as long as I wanted. Now, it's the women who sometimes ask me to take a break."*

Urologists, doctors who specialize in men's health, have known for years that the foods you eat play a key role in sexual health. As we mentioned before, the arteries that carry blood to the penis don't have a lot of surplus space. Men who eat well are less likely to accumulate arterial crud, the fatty coatings that reduce the carrying capacity of blood vessels and can make erections difficult or even impossible to achieve. At the same time, a healthful diet dramatically reduces the risk of diabetes and other chronic diseases that are among the main causes of erection problems.

Let's take a quick look at a few of them, the ones that can often be controlled with diet alone. Don't wait until next year to start. Don't even wait until tomorrow. Do it today.

▶ High cholesterol. It's among the leading causes of impotence for the simple reason that cholesterol—a waxy, fatty substance that's produced in the liver from dietary fat—often coats artery walls and greatly reduces bloodflow. Your body uses it to strengthen cell walls and produce a variety of hormones, among other things. But when the amount of cholesterol in your blood exceeds the amount your body needs, it gets deposited in the arteries. The smaller arteries, such as those in the penis, are likely to suffer first. Bigger arteries, the ones involved in heart attacks, may take decades before they accumulate enough cholesterol and other goo to cause serious problems.

It's all a lot more complicated than this, of course. There are several kinds of cholesterol, including low-density lipoprotein (LDL), the stuff that sticks like Velcro to arteries, and high-density lipoprotein (HDL), a beneficial form of cholesterol that removes LDL from the bloodstream. In terms of diet, though, the equation is straightforward: You want to avoid foods that raise LDL, while at the same time eat more of those that raise HDL.

▶ High blood pressure. The word *pressure* alone tells you that this is something you want to avoid. Too much pressure in the arteries—from smoking, eating too much salt, logging too much couch time, and so on—creates turbulence and force that literally damage and scar the artery walls. These areas of damage act like magnets for LDL cholesterol. High blood pressure increases your risk for stroke, heart attack, kidney damage, you name it. And because it's a circulatory problem, it can also wreak havoc in the bedroom.

▶ Diabetes. Most cases occur when the body's cells don't respond to insulin, the hormone that carts sugar (glucose) out of the blood and into the body's cells. This condition, called insulin resistance, causes the pancreas to churn out high amounts of insulin to overcome the resistance. Eventually, this causes the pancreas to burn out. Insulin levels drop, and blood glucose levels rise. Diabetes can damage nerves and blood vessels throughout the body and is among the leading causes of impotence in men.

Men with diabetes who improve their diets and lose weight dramatically improve—so much so that in some cases, their glucose levels return to normal. Studies show that men who lose as little as 10 percent of their weight can reduce their risk of diabetes by more than half. Even if you already have it, weight loss can reduce your need for medicine. Add some exercise to the mix, and you can lower blood glucose by 5 to 20 percent.

THE FUELS YOU NEED

Before we take a look at specific foods that have been shown to boost sexual performance, it's worth taking a quick look at the basic nutrients every man needs. If you don't get enough of these nutrients, or the mix you get is out of balance, you'll hardly have enough energy to walk to the mailbox, let alone get excited between the sheets.

Everything you eat can be divided into three main categories of *macronutrients:* protein, fats, and carbohydrates. Nutritionists have all sorts of formulas for determining your optimal intake of protein, fats, and carbohydrates. Here's the quick version. Fats, as you know, tend to contribute most to both high cholesterol and unwanted bulges around your waist. Don't eat a lot of them. Instead, focus on getting enough protein and the right kinds of carbohydrates.

▶ Protein: 33 percent of total calories. That's a rough-and-ready estimate, of course. A guy who does heavy lifting for a living might need more, while a guy who sits at a desk needs less. Protein is essential for muscle growth and development. It's involved in the manufacture of hormones, antibodies, enzymes, and tissues. It helps the body maintain the proper acid-alkali balance. And a 2000 study of 1,552 men whose mean age was 55 found that the lower their protein intake, the higher their levels of SHBG (sex hormone–binding globulin), a chemical that attaches to testosterone and keeps it from becoming available to the body. When testosterone isn't available, your body can't use it to make muscle or maintain a sex drive.

What your body really wants out of protein is the mix of amino acids it contains. You can produce some of these aminos on your own, but others can be obtained only from foods. Proteins called "complete" contain all of the amino acids that your body needs. Good sources of complete proteins include meat, fish, poultry, soy, milk, eggs, yogurt, and cheese. Proteins called "incomplete" contain some amino acids, but not all. Examples include grains, legumes, and leafy vegetables.

Meat is certainly a convenient way to fulfill your amino acid needs, but you can get the same effect by eating a wide variety of plant foods. As long as you get all of the essential amino acids that you need, it doesn't matter if they come in one tidy, T-bone package or in a variety of crunchy, leafy, grainy, or nutty things.

▼

Kissing can save you a fortune on dental bills. Deep kissing stimulates the flow of saliva, which washes away food particles and lowers levels of tooth-damaging acids in the mouth.

▲

▶ Fats: 33 percent of total calories. Fats probably have the worst rap in the food world, and in some ways, it's justified. The wrong fats— mainly the saturated fat in meats, full-fat dairy foods, and desserts, and the trans fats in margarine and hundreds of snack foods—can shoot harmful LDL cholesterol into the red zone and have been linked to colon and prostate cancers. Yet there are other fats that are more or less neutral, and some that are beneficial.

On the whole, you want to limit fat consumption to 33 percent of total calories—not only because of the direct and indirect health risks but also because fats contain about double the calories of an equal amount of protein or carbs. When you do use fats, favor the monounsaturated kinds, such as olive and canola oils. They actually elevate the beneficial form of cholesterol and can help you reduce the risk of heart disease as well as future accumulations of blood-blocking sludge in arteries in the penis and elsewhere.

▶ Carbohydrates: 33 percent of total calories. All carbohydrates are sugars. Simple carbohydrates—the fructose in fruit, the sucrose in table sugar, and the lactose in milk—are almost pure sugar. Complex carbohydrates, found in vegetables, whole grains, and legumes, consist of sugar that's strung together in more complex chains. Complex carbs are high in fiber, the indigestible stuff that lowers appetite and helps control cholesterol.

Keep in mind that carbohydrates provide the body with quick energy. They're the main source of blood glucose, a major fuel for your brain and cells. Except for the fiber component, which is impervious to human digestion, complex carbohydrates are converted into glucose, which delivers a nice, steady, energetic buzz. Compare that with straight sugar, which delivers a quick high and an equally quick crash—one that can quickly strip you of any desire to have sex. So much for topping a meal with that "romantic" dessert.

▶ Water: All you can handle. The human body is composed primarily of water. Every living cell requires water for nourishment, cooling, and the elimination of wastes. It is essential for regulation of body temperature. All vital organs need water to function at peak capacity. And research has demonstrated that proper amounts of water result in increased sex drive.

You should drink at least eight full glasses of water per day. That is the bare minimum, and it's in fact wholly insufficient for men who are in any way active. There's no perfect substitute. It's water that feeds and cleanses your cells.

If you really can't stand drinking plain water all day long, fruit juice isn't bad (see "Liquid Assets" on page 310), but it doesn't do the job as well. Coffee, tea, and even diet soda are also okay.

YOU WEAR WHAT YOU EAT

In the end, when you cut through all of the eye-glazing jargon about "fat deposition," "lipogenesis," and "The Zone," the researchers who make it their business to study this stuff come down to the same bottom line: If you take in more calories than you burn, you're going to get a bigger bottom line.

Simple.

Or maybe not. Now that more than half of Americans are overweight, and a substantial portion of those folks are obese, it's clear that the dietary advice from experts somehow isn't getting through. We're heavier than ever, and our love lives are paying the price. Men who overindulge in the kinds of foods that make you fat—beer, chips, steaks-with-everything—also have a high risk of vascular damage that inhibits bloodflow to the penis. They have a fraction of the energy of men who eat healthier foods. Then there's the visual component: A man who's way overweight isn't going to feel very confident or sexy, and the women in his life are likely to see him the same way.

This isn't the place to point fingers. We know what you need to do. You know what you need to do. You just have to decide (1) when to start taking the steps that you already know will help you lose weight and (2) how to combine the different steps in a way that's both effective and natural for your lifestyle.

If you follow even a few of the steps in this book, you'll almost automatically lose weight—without getting on and off the trend-diet bandwagon. Weight loss is simple. You have to take in fewer calories, on the one hand, and burn more calories with exercise on the other. It all boils down to a simple numbers game, with a little chemical alchemy thrown in to keep things interesting.

Figure out how much you have to lose. Standing naked in front of the mirror is a good starting place, but if you want to be a little more scientific, use a scale called the body mass index (BMI). Start with your height (in inches) and multiply that number by itself (the square). Then take your weight (in pounds) and divide it by your squared height. Finally, multiply that number by 703. That's your BMI. Or you could find it on the handy chart on the opposite page.

A BMI between 20 and 25 means you're at a healthy weight. A BMI over 25 means you have some work to do. Above 30? Get started now; you have a long way to go.

FORGET QUICK RESULTS. They're meaningless. Men who really want to drop pounds, increase energy, and improve their sex lives always do better when they lose weight slowly, about a pound or two a week. Those who jump on the latest diet bandwagons almost always fail eventually because most of these diets are so weird that no one sticks with them very long. Smart and slow beats strange and fast every time.

CUT SOME CALORIES. Since there isn't an exact number of calories that every man needs to take in each day, it's impossible to

Body Weight (lb)

Height (in)																	
58	91	96	100	105	110	115	119	124	129	134	138	143	148	153	158	162	167
59	94	99	104	109	114	119	124	128	133	138	143	148	153	158	163	168	173
60	97	102	107	112	118	123	128	133	138	143	148	153	158	163	168	174	179
61	100	106	111	116	122	127	132	137	143	148	153	158	164	169	174	180	185
62	104	109	115	120	126	131	136	142	147	153	158	164	169	175	180	186	191
63	107	113	118	124	130	135	141	146	152	158	163	169	175	180	186	191	197
64	110	116	122	128	134	140	145	151	157	163	169	174	180	186	192	197	204
65	114	120	126	132	138	144	150	156	162	168	174	180	186	192	198	204	210
66	118	124	130	136	142	148	155	161	167	173	179	186	192	198	204	210	216
67	121	127	134	140	146	153	159	166	172	178	185	191	198	204	211	217	223
68	125	131	138	144	151	158	164	171	177	184	190	197	203	210	216	223	230
69	128	135	142	149	155	162	169	176	182	189	196	203	209	216	223	230	236
70	132	139	146	153	160	167	174	181	188	195	202	209	216	222	229	236	243
71	136	143	150	157	165	172	179	186	193	200	208	215	222	229	236	243	250
72	140	147	154	162	169	177	184	191	199	206	213	221	228	235	242	250	258
73	144	151	159	166	174	182	189	197	204	212	219	227	235	242	250	257	265
74	148	155	163	171	179	186	194	202	210	218	225	233	241	249	256	264	272
75	152	160	168	176	184	192	200	208	216	224	232	240	248	256	264	272	279
76	156	164	172	180	189	197	205	213	221	230	238	246	254	263	271	279	287
BMI	19	20	21	22	23	24	25	26	27	28	29	30	31	32	33	34	35

say exactly how many you need to get rid of when you're trying to lose weight. As a general rule, cutting out 500 daily calories will cause you to lose 1 pound a week. To hit that number, though, you really have to scale back the amount you eat. It usually makes more sense to cut out some calories (say, 250 a day), and burn up some (another 250) with exercise.

SET REASONABLE GOALS. Although long-term goals such as "I want to be healthier and have better erections" are all well and good, they're not going to keep you motivated from day to day. For that you need short-term goals that are specific, realistic, achievable, and measurable.

For example, telling yourself "I will lose 3 pounds this week" is risky. After all, you might not lose the weight, and then you'll feel like you failed—and give up. A better goal would be "I will work out three times this week." That's something you can control, and doing it is a kind of reward itself. It's better to focus on what you know you can do rather than the ultimate results you hope to get.

BROADEN YOUR CONCEPT OF EXERCISE. Forget hard-core workouts for a moment. Sure, you can lose a lot of weight if you consistently work out or play tennis, but these activities account for what? A couple of hours a week? You can burn a heck of a lot of calories in the other hours just by staying active. Walking to the post office instead of driving. Finding an excuse to putter in the garden. Deliberately carrying only one or two things when you go up the stairs, so you'll have to make extra trips. Any movement increases metabolism, and calories are the fuel that keep it going. Use up the fuel, and you'll lose weight, guaranteed.

STAY ON TOP. It's worth mentioning that as a calorie-burning exercise, sex is overrated. Sure, you can burn a heck of a lot of calories, but only if you do it for a long time—longer than most of us are ready to go at any given time. Still, it's also worth mentioning that you have one big advantage over your partner—if, that is, you stay on top of the situation. You'll burn more than two times the calories per minute (5.58) when you're on top than she will on the bottom (2.5). In fact, she would burn more calories per minute if she went shopping (but don't tell her that). If you spend 10 minutes making love, and you do it twice a week, love's labors will lose you about 1½ pounds a year.

EAT SMART. Use common sense. When you're trying to lose weight, cut back on all the super-rich food in your diet: red meat, ice cream, butter, whatever. Eat more "lean" foods: rice, legumes, and fruits and vegetables. It's just another way of shaving extra calories. Take advantage of it.

STICK TO TWO A DAY. Alcohol isn't such a bad thing. Cardiologists often advise drinkers to keep it up because alcohol can

DRINKING SMART

Alcohol can certainly be part of a healthful lifestyle—cardiologists give the nod of approval to men who have a drink or two a day, because it can reduce their risk of heart disease—but it can also destroy your sexual energy if you aren't careful. Alcohol is prized as a social lubricant, and it's almost unavoidable at sports events. There aren't many alternatives to bars when you're looking to hang out with friends. Yet too many of us, especially young men, drink to reckless excess.

You need to be honest with yourself about what alcohol is and what it can do. For starters, it's a sedative, one that dampens judgment as well as inhibitions. Men who drink too much and then try to make love usually fall flat. It's worth asking yourself if alcohol allows you to do what you really want to do—or whether it entices you in directions you'd usually not go.

Too much alcohol simply isn't good for you. It kills brain cells. Excess drinking stresses the cardiovascular system. It attacks the liver. It can also damage the penis. Virtually all long-term alcoholics lose the ability to have erections. Even a single bout of heavy drinking can put you out of commission until the effects wear off.

The alcohol bottom line, as with so many other things, is that moderation has to come first. If you're a drinker, and you limit your intake to one or two drinks daily, well, keep enjoying it. Indeed, you're statistically less likely to die prematurely of a heart attack than a nondrinker. You're less likely to have a stroke. You'll probably even have less stress.

Drink more than one or two a day, however, and the benefits disappear. At that point, the risks go through the roof. It's something to think about.

dramatically reduce your risk of heart disease. The health benefits aren't so great that it's worth starting if you don't currently drink—but if you do, one or two a day can help keep the blood flowing. As long as you cut the calories from somewhere else, you can enjoy the occasional beer, glass of wine, or shot without gaining weight.

You'll notice the emphasis on "one or two." Men who drink more than that tend to have all sorts of health problems, including—but not limited to—a total inability to have sex, at least until the alcohol wears off. Then there's the small issue of weight gain: Your average 12-ounce beer has 146 calories. Multiply that by a few, and you'll understand why that spare tire is often called a beer gut.

TANK UP ON WATER. We humans, imperfect as we are, often mistake thirst for hunger. Instead of drinking some nice, clear, calorie-free water when we're feeling thirsty, we stuff our mouths with calorie-packed snacks.

The next time you feel a hankering for something, try drinking a big glass of water first. You may find that's all you really needed.

GO FOR THE GRAINS. Besides providing a lot of essential nutrients, grains are high in fiber. Fiber absorbs water like a sponge in the gut, making you feel fuller and making it easier to eat less of the kinds of things that pack on the pounds. The even better thing about fiber is that it essentially yanks cholesterol out of your blood before it has a chance to jam the essential blood vessels that fuel erections.

EAT MORE BEANS. It's true that some beans, like pintos, are powerful little gas grenades, but don't let that stop you. Beans are among the most nutritious foods you can eat, and they're filling. More beans means less steak, ice cream, and all of that other rich stuff that sends the scale into the red zone. And because beans are high in fiber, they'll help keep blood circulating when you need it most.

GIVE IT A TRIM. If your idea of a three-course meal is to have a couple of beers with your steak, at least do this: Trim away the excess fat before you put that New York strip on the grill. Each of those fat grams has about nine calories, double what you'll get from the same amount of baked potato. To make life easier, chill the meat for about 20 minutes. The fat will turn white, making it easier to see. Plus, the meat will firm up a bit, making it easier to trim.

DON'T STOCK IT. The "it" refers to doughnuts, chips, and all of those other delicious, put-on-the-pounds snacks that are simply too hard to resist if you have them in the house. The Food Cops won't bust you when you shovel in the occasional Krispy Kreme or bury your hand in the bowl of beer nuts at the bar. But if you keep too many snacks in the house where they're easy to get to, you're going to eat them, probably all at once.

LET FORTUNE BE YOUR GUIDE. When you go out to eat, celebrate. Want that fancy single malt? Have it. Enjoy. The steak smothered in mushrooms? Life is short; dig in. The reason so many men crash off their diets is that they're forced to give up everything good. Don't let it happen to you. Eat well most days, keep your larder stocked with things you know are healthy, and then have a good time when you go out. You'll feel rewarded (and stuffed), and you'll be more likely to stick with the plan the rest of the time.

PICK YOUR BATTLES. High-calorie fat and sugar are in just about anything you eat—certainly anything that comes in a box or off a fast-food line. Even an apple, innocent as it looks, hides inside itself about half a gram of fat. So do you become paranoid? Obsessive? Start counting every gram you eat?

Not at all. You can lop a lot of calories from your diet just by changing a few of your worst habits—like the daily Butterfinger bar, the dollop of butter on your potato, the Double Whopper with cheese.

The idea isn't to give up everything but to give up the things that aren't really important to you. In other words, get rid of the expendable stuff, while hanging onto the foods you really, really like. Some men, for example, have to have butter on their corn. Others don't care about that, but they have to have ice cream a few times a week. Pick your favorites, keep them, and discard the rest.

In other words, don't become a weight-loss zealot, or you'll just end up hating your life—and will almost certainly gain all the weight back. Instead, look for daily opportunities to shun calories and substitute a few healthier habits for the bad ones.

FOODS FOR SEX

You can make nutrition as complicated as you like, but for practical purposes, it's not much more complicated than we've described. If you follow the basics—keeping your weight down, eating less junk food, and getting the right mix of protein, carbs, and fats—you're going to have more energy than you did before. Simple as that.

Energy, of course, is one thing, and sexual energy and capacity are something else altogether. Which brings us to the subject of food and sex. In the past few decades, researchers have gotten pretty good at decoding the chemical mix in the foods we eat. What they've discovered is that most plant foods—beans, grains, salads, all that—contain hundreds of chemical compounds that have very specific, and sometimes sex-enhancing, effects.

They're not aphrodisiacs, in the sense of driving up libido and inflaming desire. Rather, many of these chemicals essentially fine-tune the machinery of sex by reducing cholesterol buildup and enhancing bloodflow, stimulating the release of feel-good brain chemicals and hormones, and giving cells in the penis and elsewhere the chemical energy they need to work at top capacity.

Consider carrots—and forget their suggestive shape. That vibrant orange color is produced by beta-carotene, a plant compound that reduces buildups of LDL cholesterol in the arteries and may make it easier for men to get and sustain erections. Beta-carotene isn't the only chemical that does this. It belongs to an enormous chemical family called carotenoids. These, along with hundreds of other phytochemicals, have a variety of male-protecting benefits. For example:

▶ Carotenoids essentially neutralize free radicals, harmful oxygen molecules in the body that damage cholesterol and make it more likely to stick to artery walls in the penis, heart, and other parts of the body.

▶ Some carotenoids, such as the lycopene in tomatoes, reduce the risk of prostate cancer, one of the leading sex-killers in men.

▶ The flavonoids in apples, onions, and berries act like a Teflon coating for the millions of tiny disks in your blood called platelets. The more slippery these platelets, the lower your risk of getting blood clots in the arteries.

▶ The allylic sulfides in garlic and onions do more than make your eyes water. They help keep the arteries flexible and may promote better bloodflow to the penis. At the same time, they help prevent cholesterol from jamming the tiny pipes that make erections possible.

These examples just scratch the surface, but they give a sense of what you can achieve with diet alone—and not a strange diet, either. You don't have to dig through produce bins for brown, knobby foods with unfamiliar names. Just about all of the fruits, vegetables, and other produce you can think of contain a variety of these chemicals, along with basic vitamins and minerals that you need to stay active.

Obviously, different foods supply different things. An orange will give a good dose of vitamin C, but no vitamin B_{12}. A hunk of cheese will give you B_{12}, but no vitamin C. Which is why the first rule of good nutrition, especially when you're eating for sexual health, is to eat the widest possible range of foods.

Which are best? Well, they're *all* good, but some foods seem to give the biggest bang in terms of sexual performance, endurance, fertility, and more. Many are plant based; others are the kinds of mouth-watering favorites that you slap on the grill or dish up with a spoon. If you tweak your diet today, you could be having the best sex of your life tomorrow—and every day after that.

TURN UP THE HEAT WITH ASPARAGUS. These brilliant green spears are loaded with potassium, phosphorus, calcium, and vitamin E, key nutrients for energy and urinary health. They also provide the nutrients your body needs to produce testosterone and other sex hormones.

HEAT UP WITH CHILES. They contain capsaicin, a chemical compound that causes your heart to race and your skin to flush—a sure sign that bloodflow is on the fast track. They dilate blood vessels and help all of that blood get where it's needed.

DE-STRESS WITH EGGS. Every man gets a little nervous when he's with a new partner, and that nervousness can, well, you know. A plateful of eggs in the morning can help because they're high in B vitamins, nutrients that help reduce anxiety—and get depleted during high-stress times. The B vitamins have also been shown to help keep libido high.

It turns out real men *should* eat quiche. The eggs and milk make it high in protein, which helps control SHBG—a substance that makes it harder for your body to use testosterone and arginine. Arginine is an amino acid that improves the flow of blood to the penis and may improve sexual stamina for both men and women. Go ahead and add some asparagus and potatoes to the quiche: They contain magnesium and potassium, minerals that help prevent an ill-timed charley horse from putting a damper on your fun.

GET HER HOT WITH CHOCOLATE. There's a good reason women often call it the love food. The cocoa in chocolate contains stimulants that increase skin sensitivity. Chocolate also contains compounds that are chemically similar to the euphoria-inducing hormone your body produces when you're in love.

CIRCULATE WITH OATS. It's hard to think of anything less sexy than a bowl of mushy oatmeal—but the benefits of oats can be very sexy indeed. Oats contain a variety of compounds that aid circulation and prevent cholesterol buildup. The primary ones are tocotrienols, related to vitamin E but 50 percent more powerful. As with other complex carbohydrates, oats can help reduce nervous anxiety. And they're high in fiber, the tough plant stuff that lowers cholesterol and helps maintain bloodflow.

▼

> "A man too busy to take care of his health is like a mechanic too busy to take care of his tools."
> —SPANISH PROVERB

▲

GET THE PEANUT PAYOFF. These crunchy nuts, roasted or plain, are rich in arginine, an amino acid that dilates blood vessels and promotes better erections.

FISH FOR BETTER SEX. Yep, caviar, oysters, lobster, and other delicacies from the sea deserve their sexy reputations. They're loaded with zinc, the mineral that increases the production of testosterone and promotes male fertility and prostate health.

SUCK DOWN SOME CITRUS. Nearly all fresh and frozen fruits are high in vitamin C; oranges, grapefruit, and other citrus fruits are C standouts. University of Texas researchers report that men who get at least 200 milligrams of vitamin C a day have higher sperm counts than those who consume less. Vitamin C also keeps your sperm from clumping, so your boys have a better chance of hitting pay dirt.

MUNCH A STALK. True, celery is about as bland and flavorless as a food can be, but consider this: It contains androsterone, a powerful male hormone that is released through sweat and potentially acts as a pheromone—a scent molecule that taps into the primitive part of the brain and attracts members of the opposite sex.

SPOON UP ENDURANCE. The age-old argument about the respective merits of chocolate and vanilla ice cream is now settled: Go for the white stuff. Any ice cream is good, as long as it's low-fat, because it's high in calcium and phosphorus, minerals that build muscular energy reserves and boost libido. All of that calcium can also make orgasms more powerful since the muscles that control ejaculation need calcium in order to contract properly.

Why vanilla over, say, Cherry Garcia? A study conducted at Chicago's Smell and Taste Treatment and Research Foundation found that when men smell the scent of vanilla, it relaxes them and reduces anxiety and inhibitions.

SAY "NUTS" TO INFERTILITY. All sorts of environmental toxins, including cigarette smoke and air pollution, can damage sperm and increase the risk of birth defects. Brazil nuts are a top source of selenium, a mineral that helps keep sperm cells healthy while also helping them swim faster. United Kingdom researchers report that men with fertility problems who increase their selenium intake have hardier, more viable sperm. Brazil nuts are also high in vitamin E, an antioxidant that helps protect sperm cells from free-radical damage.

BOOST SPERM WITH LIVER. It doesn't sound sexy, but ounce for ounce, there are few better sources of fertility-boosting vitamin A than liver. Studies show that men who get plenty of A each day have higher sperm counts and perform better sexually than men who don't. Liver is also an excellent source of zinc. Your body expels 5 milligrams of zinc—a third of your daily requirement—every time you ejaculate, so a single amorous weekend could leave your body's zinc reserves on empty.

SHAKE HER TREE WITH PEACHES. Oranges get the good press as a vitamin C source, but frozen peaches are a better choice. That's important if you're looking to add some deductions to your 1040, because men who don't take in enough vitamin C produce lower-quality sperm.

Keep a bag of frozen peach slices—they have more C than fresh ones do—in your freezer to dump in smoothies or add to your morning cereal. A single cup of the fruit has more than twice your daily vitamin C requirement.

GET BETTER ERECTIONS WITH BLUEBERRIES. Forget Viagra. Mother Nature's original blue potency capsules may do even more for you. Blueberries are high in soluble fiber, which helps remove excess cholesterol from the blood before it gets absorbed and deposited on artery walls. Blueberries also relax blood vessels and improve bloodflow. What that means, of course, is that more blood enters the penis to produce stronger erections. For maximum potency and performance, eat a serving of blueberries at least three or four times a week.

PUT SNAP, CRACKLE, AND POP IN YOUR SEX LIFE. Too tired for sex? Check the label on your morning cereal and make sure that you're eating a brand that's loaded with thiamin and riboflavin. Both vitamins help you use energy efficiently, so you'll stop falling asleep in the recliner while watching *Everybody Loves Raymond.* You need these nutrients for your nervous system to function efficiently. Better nerve function means more stimulation and pleasure during sex.

It's especially important to get more of these nutrients as you get older, because your body has a harder time absorbing them. Fortified breads and cereals are also high in niacin, a vitamin that's essential for the secretion of histamine, a chemical your body needs in order to trigger explosive orgasms.

EAT STEAK TO KEEP YOUR RELATIONSHIP SIZZLING.
Sparks can dwindle after you've been with the same person for a long time. An easy way to reignite them? Visit your favorite steak house and order up some lean sirloin. The protein in steak will naturally boost levels of dopamine and norepinephrine, two chemicals in the brain that heighten sensitivity during sex.

Steak is also stuffed with zinc, the mineral that boosts libido by reducing your body's production of a hormone called prolactin, which may interfere with arousal. And best of all, eating red meat can help boost your testosterone level while limiting your body's production of SHBG, which prevents bloodflow to the penis and reduces male sexual stamina.

SUCK DOWN THE OJ. If you don't have enough beneficial HDL cholesterol scouring your arteries, even low amounts of harmful LDL can form blockages that could reduce your ability to have erections. The higher the HDL, the better. Once you get more than 60 milligrams per deciliter of blood, it can help protect your heart as well. One of the best ways to boost HDL is to drink at least three glasses of OJ a week—along with running or fast-walking at least 7 miles a week and dropping at least 10 pounds if you're overweight.

HAVE A GLASS OF LOW-FAT MOO. Dairy's a great source of protein and riboflavin. The calcium in low-fat milk and cheese, apart from strengthening bones, has a little bonus: Muscles use it to contract, and getting enough calcium can make orgasms better and stronger. You also need this mineral to increase muscular energy and maintain a strong sex drive.

HAVE AN APPLE A DAY. Eating apples can reduce the artery-clogging cholesterol that can impair bloodflow to your penis—and may affect her sexual response as well. Apples contain phenylalanine, an amino acid that increases the production of endorphins, brain chemicals that may fuel sexual arousal.

SPICE IT UP WITH CINNAMON. Researchers at Chicago's Smell and Taste Treatment and Research Foundation noted an increased number of erections in men who sniffed the spice.

THE *BUILT FOR SEX* EATING PLAN

The following 7-day menu plan was designed with your sex life in mind. Based on a macronutrient content of 33 percent protein, 33 percent carbohydrates, and 33 percent fats, it's got real, guy-friendly foods with good-quality fats to help keep your arteries open—remember, good sex is all about bloodflow. Plus, the plan includes the foods and nutrients that offer you palpable sexual benefits. (Check the parentheses after each food item to see what makes it so potent.)

Each daily menu offers a total of about 2,000 calories, from which you can either add or subtract calories depending on your needs. These 2,000 calories are the *basis* for your personalized plan, which you will figure out based on your metabolism, activity level, weight, age, and goals.

Once you do the calculations on the following pages, you'll know your caloric starting point. If it turns out you need 2,500 calories a day just to maintain a healthy weight, simply add 500 calories to the plan from the "Customize It" list for each day. If you need to lose weight, adjust the plan accordingly. Simply reduce the total number of calories you eat in a day by 300 to 500 to drop about a pound a week. (The amount you lose will vary depending on your starting weight, how many calories you cut, how much you exercise, and your metabolism.) Again, the "Customize It" list included with each day's menu will give you an idea of what you can cut out to reduce calories. The comprehensive food list starting on page 343 provides calorie counts for all the foods in the plan.

To personalize the plan, start by using the following equation to figure out how many calories it takes for you to keep your body the way it is right now.

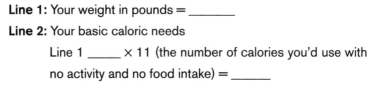

Line 1: Your weight in pounds = _____

Line 2: Your basic caloric needs

Line 1 _____ × 11 (the number of calories you'd use with no activity and no food intake) = _____

You probably do more than just laze around on the couch avoiding food. That's why you also need to factor in the effect your activity level has on your metabolism. Which of the following three activity levels describes you best?

1. Sedentary. You have a desk job, don't exercise regularly, and don't have hobbies or other activities that keep you on your feet.

2. Moderately active. You spend at least 2 hours a day on your feet, whether for work or play, or you have a daily hour-long exercise routine.

3. Dedicated exerciser/athlete. You do a high-intensity exercise almost every day, or you've been lifting weights 3 or 4 days a week for at least a year. A weight lifter's metabolism burns calories at a relatively high rate even at rest because of his muscle mass. The guy who plays basketball or hockey regularly burns up a lot of calories simply from the activity itself.

Age also makes a difference in your metabolic factor. Everyone starts to slow down after adolescence—it's part of the normal aging process. Once you hit age 30, inactivity slows your metabolic rate by about 1 percent a year. It's possible to reverse this at any age with muscle-building exercise. Here are some figures to start with.

	YOUNGER THAN 30	30–40 YEARS OLD	OLDER THAN 40
Sedentary	30%	25%	20%
Moderately active	40%	35%	30%
Dedicated exerciser/athlete	50%	45%	40%

Multiply the appropriate percentage by your basic calorie needs to calculate your metabolic factor.

Line 3: Your metabolic factor

Line 2 _____ × _____% = _____

Now you can figure out the number of calories you need to maintain the status quo. Add your basic calorie needs to your metabolic factor.

Line 4: Your maintenance diet

Line 2 _____ + Line 3 _____ = _____

The final factor for determining how to use the *Built for Sex* Eating Plan is your goals. Do you want to maintain your weight, gain, or lose? Since a pound of fat equals 3,500 calories, you'll need to add or subtract 500 calories a day to gain or lose a pound a week. Example: Say you're a 45-year-old, 230-pound guy, and you want to lose weight. You're sedentary now, so your metabolic factor is 20 percent, which brings you to a 3,000-calorie-per-day maintenance diet. Subtract 500 calories (to get to 2,500 calories a day), and lose 1 pound a week.

What if you're a very active 150-pound 25-year-old who wants to gain muscle weight? Simply add 500 calories to a 2,475-calorie-a-day diet, and you get about 3,000 calories (rounded up). You should gain about a pound of muscle a week by eating that many daily calories.

Finally, say you're a 35-year-old, 180-pound guy who's fairly active and doesn't want to gain or lose weight—just maybe shave an inch off the waistline and add some muscle to your chest and shoulders. Do the math for a maintenance calorie intake of about 2,700 daily calories.

One caveat: Try to keep your calorie intake at 2,000 or above even if your calculations indicate you need fewer. Eating less than that can compromise your testosterone levels and your ability to build muscle, sabotaging your quest for a more satisfying sex life.

Of course, any time you change your eating regimen, you should consult your doctor. And if you have kidney disease, consult your physician before starting any diet high in protein.

What do you drink with these meals, you ask? Try water, unsweetened iced tea, or diet soda.

THE MENUS

❶ DAY ONE

Breakfast

1½ cups whole grain, high-fiber cereal (thiamin, riboflavin, niacin)

1 cup 1% milk (calcium, riboflavin, vitamins A and D)

3 links turkey sausage (zinc, iron, arginine, niacin, vitamins B_6 and B_{12})

½ cup fresh pineapple chunks (vitamin C, potassium)

Snack

Ham and cheese rollup made with

4 oz lean deli ham (zinc, iron, arginine, thiamin, riboflavin, niacin, vitamins B_6 and B_{12})

1 oz low-fat Swiss cheese (calcium, vitamin B_{12}, zinc)

1 small apple, chopped (flavonoids, potassium)

Lunch

Roast beef sandwich made with

5 oz lean roast beef (zinc, iron, arginine, riboflavin, niacin, vitamins B_6 and B_{12})

2 slices low-carb bread

1 Tbsp Miracle Whip

2 Tbsp horseradish

2 slices tomato (lycopene, vitamin C, potassium)

Romaine lettuce (carotenoids, folate, vitamin B_6)

Snack

2 oz low-fat string cheese (calcium, vitamin B_{12})

1 cup 1% milk (calcium, riboflavin, vitamins A and D)

Dinner

4 oz baked salmon (arginine, omega-3 fatty acids, vitamin B_{12})

1 small sweet potato (4 oz), baked (beta-carotene, vitamins E, C, and B_6)

2 cups spinach (beta-carotene, folate, iron, potassium, magnesium, vitamins B_6 and C) sautéed in 1½ tsp olive oil (vitamin E)

Dessert

½ cup low-fat vanilla bean ice cream (calcium, phosphorus, riboflavin)

1 Tbsp low-calorie dark chocolate syrup (methylxanthines, phenylethylamine)

1 Tbsp dry-roasted, unsalted peanuts, crushed (arginine, vitamin E, magnesium, niacin)

Nutritional analysis: 2,066 calories, 174 grams (g) carbohydrates, 177 g protein, 78 g fat, 20 g sat fat, 369 milligrams (mg) cholesterol, 25 g fiber, 3,845 mg sodium

▶CUSTOMIZE IT

ADD CALORIES	SUBTRACT CALORIES
1 cup low-fat plain or vanilla yogurt (155)	3 oz low-fat cheese (150)
1 small banana (80)	4 oz lean deli ham (120)
1 oz almonds (170)	½ cup low-fat vanilla bean ice cream (90)
1 cup orange juice (110)	1 Tbsp low-calorie dark chocolate syrup (25)
1 roast beef sandwich (535)	1 Tbsp dry-roasted, unsalted peanuts, crushed (50)

❷DAY TWO

Breakfast

Wrap made with

> 2 scrambled eggs (B vitamins, iron, zinc)
>
> ⅓ cup chopped red and green bell peppers (lycopene, capsaicin, vitamin C) sautéed in 1 tsp soft canola margarine
>
> ½ cup spicy salsa (lycopene, vitamin C, potassium, capsaicin)
>
> 1 whole grain tortilla (8") (B vitamins)

1 cup 1% milk (calcium, riboflavin, vitamins A and D)

Snack

1 cup low-fat plain or vanilla yogurt (calcium, phosphorus)

½ cup fresh blueberries (vitamin C)

Lunch

Sandwich made with

> 5 oz turkey breast (zinc, iron, arginine, niacin, vitamins B_6 and B_{12})
>
> 2 oz low-fat Swiss cheese (calcium, vitamin B_{12}, zinc)
>
> 2 slices low-carb bread
>
> 1 Tbsp Miracle Whip
>
> 2 Tbsp mashed avocado (beta-carotene, potassium)
>
> 2 slices tomato (lycopene, vitamin C, potassium)
>
> Watercress sprigs (carotenoids, folate, iron, potassium, vitamins B_6 and C)

Snack

2 oz low-fat Cheddar cheese (calcium, vitamin B$_{12}$)

1 oz sesame seed breadsticks (B vitamins, calcium, magnesium, selenium)

Dinner

2 lean pork chops, grilled (7 oz) (protein, zinc, iron, arginine, thiamin, other B vitamins)

½ cup vegetarian baked beans (iron, potassium, phosphorus, magnesium)

1 cup sliced carrots, lightly steamed (beta-carotene) with 1 tsp soft canola margarine

½ cup fresh mango cubes (beta-carotene, vitamin C, potassium)

Nutritional analysis: 2,090 calories, 174 g carbohydrates, 174 g protein, 80 g fat, 22 g sat fat, 616 mg cholesterol, 26 g fiber, 3,007 mg sodium

▶CUSTOMIZE IT

ADD CALORIES	SUBTRACT CALORIES
1 whole grain English muffin (135)	3 oz low-fat cheese (150)
2 Tbsp peanut butter (190)	1 oz sesame seed breadsticks (120)
1 small apple (60)	1 whole grain tortilla (8") (160)
1 cup 1% milk (100)	1 tsp soft canola margarine (35)
1 turkey, Swiss, and avocado sandwich (540)	

❸DAY THREE

Breakfast

1 cup old-fashioned oatmeal (tocotrienols) topped with

    1 tsp ground flaxseed (lignans, omega-3 fatty acids)

    1 tsp cinnamon and brown sugar

    ½ cup 1% milk (calcium, riboflavin, vitamins A and D)

4 links turkey sausage (zinc, iron, arginine, niacin, vitamins B$_6$ and B$_{12}$)

Snack

½ cup canned unsweetened sliced peaches (vitamin C, potassium)

1 cup 1% cottage cheese (calcium, magnesium, phosphorus, potassium, selenium)

Lunch

Sandwich made with

   2 oz low-fat Cheddar cheese (calcium, vitamin B_{12})

   2 slices low-carb bread

   1 Tbsp Miracle Whip

   2 Tbsp spicy mustard

   2 slices tomato (lycopene, vitamin C, potassium)

   Spinach (beta-carotene, folate, iron, potassium, magnesium, vitamins B_6 and C)

1 small ripe banana (potassium)

1 cup 1% milk (calcium, riboflavin, vitamins A and D)

Snack

3.5 oz canned smoked oysters (arginine, iron, selenium, zinc, vitamin B_{12})

4 saltine crackers (B vitamins)

1 oz dry-roasted, unsalted peanuts (arginine, vitamin E, magnesium, niacin)

Dinner

6 oz skinless chicken breast, grilled (zinc, arginine, niacin, B vitamins) brushed with 2 Tbsp barbecue sauce

⅓ cup brown rice pilaf

1½ cups olive-oil roasted vegetables (beta-carotene, potassium, vitamins C and E)

½ medium grapefruit (lycopene, vitamin C)

Nutritional analysis: 2,092 calories, 181 g carbohydrates, 178 g protein, 77 g fat, 19 g sat fat, 341 mg cholesterol, 29 g fiber, 4,084 mg sodium

▶CUSTOMIZE IT

ADD CALORIES	SUBTRACT CALORIES
1 peanut butter smoothie (350)	1 cup 1% cottage cheese (160)
1 medium (1 oz) oatmeal-raisin cookie (125)	4 saltine crackers (50)
1 hard-cooked egg (75)	1 oz dry-roasted, unsalted peanuts (165)
1 cheese sandwich (350)	2 turkey sausage links (90)

④ DAY FOUR

Breakfast

2 soft-boiled eggs (B vitamins, iron, zinc)

2 slices whole grain bread (B vitamins)

2 slices Canadian bacon (zinc, iron, arginine, thiamin, other B vitamins)

1 cup low-calorie cranberry juice (flavonoids, ellagic acid, vitamin C)

2 fat-free Fig Newtons (potassium, vitamin B_6)

1 cup 1% milk (calcium, riboflavin, vitamins A and D)

1 oz Brazil nuts (selenium, vitamin E, arginine, calcium, magnesium)

Lunch

Salad made with

2 oz turkey breast strips (zinc, iron, arginine, niacin, B vitamins)

3 oz lean deli ham strips (zinc, iron, arginine, thiamin, other B vitamins)

2 oz low-fat Swiss cheese strips (calcium, vitamin B_{12})

2 cups mixed salad greens (carotenoids, folate, vitamin B_6, vitamin C, iron, potassium)

½ cup grated carrot (beta-carotene)

½ cup sliced cucumber (potassium)

¼ cup reduced-fat creamy dressing

Snack

1 oz low-fat string cheese (calcium, vitamin B_{12})

1 cup 1% chocolate milk (methylxanthines, phenylethylamine, calcium, riboflavin, vitamins A and D)

Dinner

2 lean lamb chops (7 oz), grilled (zinc, iron, B vitamins)

2 small (5 oz) red potatoes, baked (potassium, vitamin C)

½ cup spicy salsa (lycopene, vitamin C, potassium, capsaicin)

8 asparagus spears, steamed (potassium, phosphorus, calcium, vitamin E) with 1 tsp soft canola margarine

½ cup canned unsweetened pears

Nutritional analysis: 2,072 calories, 173 g carbohydrates, 170 g protein, 78 g fat, 22 g sat fat, 699 mg cholesterol, 20 g fiber, 4,871 mg sodium

▶CUSTOMIZE IT

ADD CALORIES	SUBTRACT CALORIES
⅓ cup granola (180)	2 fat-free Fig Newtons (130)
1 oz raisins (85)	2 oz low-fat cheese (100)
1 oz almonds (170)	1 cup 1% chocolate milk(180)
1 cup unsweetened apple juice (110)	1 tsp soft canola margarine (35)
1 turkey, ham, and Swiss cheese salad (395)	

❺DAY FIVE

Breakfast

2 whole grain waffles (4") (B vitamins, calcium, magnesium, phosphorus) with 2 Tbsp light pancake syrup

1 cup low-fat plain or vanilla yogurt (calcium, phosphorus)

½ cup canned unsweetened sliced peaches (vitamin C, potassium)

1 cup 1% milk (calcium, riboflavin, vitamins A and D)

Snack

1 oz raisins (potassium, iron)

1 oz sunflower or pumpkin seeds (zinc, magnesium, vitamin E)

Lunch

Sandwich made with

> 1 can (7 oz) water-packed chunk white tuna (iron, arginine, selenium, vitamin B_{12})
>
> 2 slices low-carb bread
>
> 1 Tbsp Miracle Whip
>
> 2 slices tomato (lycopene, vitamin C, potassium)
>
> Romaine lettuce (carotenoids, folate, vitamin B_6)

1 can (6 oz) spicy V-8 (lycopene, vitamin C, potassium)

1 oz low-fat string cheese (calcium, riboflavin, vitamin B_{12})

Snack

¼ cup garlicky hummus (iron, potassium, phosphorus, magnesium, allylic sulfides)

1 stalk celery (androsterone, androstenol)

1 hard-cooked egg (B vitamins, iron, zinc)

Dinner

6 oz baked cod or halibut (arginine, vitamin B_{12}) seasoned with cayenne pepper (capsaicin)

½ cup cooked whole wheat pasta

½ cup marinara sauce (lycopene, vitamin C, potassium)

2 cups spinach or collards (beta-carotene, folate, iron, potassium, vitamins B_6 and C) sautéed in 1 tsp olive oil and garlic (vitamin E, allylic sulfides)

½ cup fresh cantaloupe cubes (beta-carotene, vitamin C, potassium)

Nutritional analysis: 2,092 calories, 178 g carbohydrates, 179 g protein, 78 g fat, 16 g sat fat, 454 mg cholesterol, 22 g fiber, 3,629 mg sodium

▶CUSTOMIZE IT

ADD CALORIES	SUBTRACT CALORIES
1 slice whole wheat raisin bread (75)	2 Tbsp light pancake syrup (50)
¼ cup part-skim ricotta cheese with 4 slices kiwifruit (100)	1 cup low-fat plain or vanilla yogurt (155)
1 cup 1% milk (100)	1 slice low-carb bread (85)
1 oz walnuts (185)	¼ cup hummus (100)
1 tuna sandwich (455)	1 oz low-fat cheese (50)

❻DAY SIX

Breakfast

1 cup whole grain, high-fiber cereal (thiamin, riboflavin, niacin)

¼ cup fresh blueberries (vitamin C)

1 cup 1% milk (calcium, riboflavin, vitamins A and D)

2 links turkey sausage (zinc, iron, arginine, niacin, vitamins B_6 and B_{12})

Snack

1 slice low-carb bread

2 Tbsp low-fat cream cheese (calcium, phosphorus)

Lunch

Chicken salad sandwich made with

6 oz grilled chicken, cubed (zinc, arginine, niacin, other B vitamins)

1 cup spinach leaves (beta-carotene, folate, iron, potassium, vitamins B_6 and C)

½ cup grated carrot (beta-carotene)

¼ cup chopped red and green bell peppers
(lycopene, capsaicin, vitamin C)

6 walnuts (arginine, vitamin E, magnesium, omega-3 fatty acids)

½ cup chopped apple (flavonoids, potassium)

1 whole wheat pita (6½") (B vitamins)

¼ cup reduced-fat creamy dressing

Snack

2 oz low-fat string cheese (calcium, vitamin B_{12})

1 cup 1% milk (calcium, riboflavin, vitamins A and D)

Dinner

6 oz lean flank steak, grilled (zinc, iron, arginine, B vitamins)

1 cup steamed broccoli, cauliflower, and zucchini (beta-carotene,
vitamin C) with 1 tsp soft canola margarine

1 whole grain roll (B vitamins) with 1 tsp soft canola margarine

½ cup red seedless grapes (flavonoids, potassium)

Nutritional analysis: 2,055 calories, 174 g carbohydrates, 175 g protein, 76 g fat, 23 g sat fat, 347 mg cholesterol, 25 g fiber, 3,145 mg sodium

▶CUSTOMIZE IT

ADD CALORIES	SUBTRACT CALORIES
1 peach (60)	1 slice low-carb bread (85)
3 (1 oz) gingersnaps (90)	2 Tbsp low-fat cream cheese (70)
1 cup 1% chocolate milk (180)	2 oz low-fat cheese (100)
½ whole grain English muffin (70)	1 whole wheat pita (6½") (170)
1 Tbsp apple butter (30)	1 tsp soft canola margarine (35)
1 chicken salad sandwich in pita (570)	

❼ DAY SEVEN

Breakfast

Omelet made with

  2 scrambled eggs (B vitamins, iron, zinc)

  2 oz low-fat cheese, shredded (calcium, vitamin B_{12})

  ½ cup asparagus tips (potassium, phosphorus, calcium, vitamin E) sautéed in 1 tsp soft canola margarine

2 slices Canadian bacon (zinc, iron, arginine, thiamin, B vitamins)

1 whole wheat pita (6½") (B vitamins)

1 cup orange juice (vitamin C, potassium)

Snack

1 cup tomato-basil soup, made with 1% milk (lycopene, vitamin C, potassium)

4 saltine crackers (B vitamins)

Lunch

Antipasto salad made with

  3 oz turkey breast (zinc, iron, arginine, niacin, B vitamins)

  2 oz low-fat Colby cheese (calcium, vitamin B_{12})

  6 green olives (vitamin E)

  4 marinated artichoke hearts (potassium)

  ½ roasted red pepper (lycopene, vitamin C)

1 whole grain roll (B vitamins)

Snack

Peanut butter smoothie made with

  1 cup 1% milk (calcium, riboflavin, vitamins A and D)

  1 cup thawed frozen strawberries (anthocyanins, ellagic acid, vitamin C)

  2 Tbsp peanut butter (arginine, vitamin E, magnesium, niacin)

Dinner

6 oz skinless chicken breast, roasted (zinc, arginine, niacin, B vitamins)

1 medium ear corn with 1 tsp soft canola margarine

1 cup green beans, steamed (carotenoids, calcium, potassium) with 1 Tbsp slivered almonds (vitamin E, arginine, calcium, magnesium) and 1 tsp soft canola margarine

1 slice watermelon, 1" × 10" (lycopene)

Nutritional analysis: 2,035 calories, 174 g carbohydrates, 170 g protein, 76 g fat, 22 g sat fat, 667 mg cholesterol, 24 g fiber, 4,665 mg sodium

▶CUSTOMIZE IT

ADD CALORIES	SUBTRACT CALORIES
1 oz dry-roasted, unsalted peanuts (165)	1 oz low-fat cheese (50)
1 small banana (80)	1 whole grain roll (80)
1 cup 1% milk (100)	1 peanut butter smoothie (350)
1 cheese sandwich (350)	

BUILT FOR SEX FOODS AT A GLANCE

This comprehensive list includes all the foods in the *Built for Sex* Eating Plan. These are the sexiest, healthiest foods on the planet. Photocopy this list and take it with you to the supermarket. Food shopping has never been so easy.

BREADS, CEREALS, AND GRAINS

1 slice whole grain bread (80 calories)

1 slice whole wheat raisin bread (75)

1 slice low-carb bread (85)

1 whole grain roll (80)

1 whole grain English muffin (135)

1 whole wheat pita (6½") (170)

1 whole grain tortilla (8") (160)

1 oz. sesame seed breadsticks (120)

2 saltine crackers (25)

1 cup old-fashioned oatmeal (145)

⅓ cup granola (180)

1 cup whole grain, high-fiber cereal (150)

2 whole grain waffles (4") (210)

⅓ cup brown rice pilaf (85)

½ cup cooked whole wheat pasta (80)

DAIRY PRODUCTS AND EGGS

1 egg, scrambled, soft-boiled, or hard-cooked (75)

1 cup 1% milk (100)

1 cup 1% chocolate milk (180)

1 oz low-fat cheese (all types) (50)

1 cup 1% cottage cheese (160)

2 Tbsp low-fat cream cheese (70)

¼ cup part-skim ricotta cheese (45)

1 cup low-fat plain or vanilla yogurt (155)

CONDIMENTS AND DRESSINGS

2 Tbsp barbecue sauce (70)

2 Tbsp horseradish (15)

1 Tbsp spicy mustard (10)

¼ cup reduced-fat creamy dressing (100)

½ cup spicy salsa (35)

FATS, NUTS, AND OILS

1 oz almonds (170)

1 oz Brazil nuts (195)

1 tsp ground flaxseed (25)

1 Tbsp peanut butter (95)

1 oz dry-roasted, unsalted peanuts (165)

1 Tbsp dry-roasted, unsalted peanuts, crushed (50)

1 oz pumpkin seeds (150)

1 oz sunflower seeds (140)

1 oz walnuts (185)

2 Tbsp mashed avocado (45)

1 tsp canola soft margarine (35)

1 Tbsp Miracle Whip (70)

1 Tbsp olive oil (110)

6 green olives (65)

FRUITS

1 small apple (60)

1 Tbsp apple butter (30)

1 cup unsweetened apple juice (110)

1 small banana (80)

½ cup fresh blueberries (40)

½ cup fresh cantaloupe cubes (40)

1 cup low-calorie cranberry juice (45)

1 oz dried figs (70)

½ cup seedless grapes (30)

½ medium grapefruit (60)

4 slices kiwifruit (15)

½ cup fresh mango (60)

1 cup orange juice (110)

1 small peach (60)

½ cup canned unsweetened sliced peaches (60)

½ cup canned unsweetened pears (80)

½ cup fresh pineapple chunks (40)

1 oz raisins (85)

1 cup thawed frozen strawberries (60)

1 slice watermelon, 1" × 10" (130)

MEATS, POULTRY, AND SEAFOOD

1 oz lean flank steak (45)

1 slice Canadian bacon (40)

1 oz skinless chicken or turkey breast (30)

1 oz cod or halibut (30)

1 oz lean sliced deli ham (30)

1 oz lean lamb (40)

1 oz canned smoked oysters (25)

1 oz lean pork (35)

1 oz lean roast beef (55)

1 oz salmon (50)

1 oz water-packed chunk white tuna (30)

1 turkey sausage link (45)

SNACKS AND DESSERTS

1 tsp brown sugar (15)

1 Tbsp low-calorie dark chocolate syrup (25)

2 Tbsp light pancake syrup (50)

2 fat-free Fig Newtons (130)

3 (1 oz) gingersnaps (90)

1 medium (1 oz) oatmeal-raisin cookie (125)

½ cup low-fat vanilla bean ice cream (90)

VEGETABLES

1 marinated artichoke heart (15)

4 asparagus spears, cooked (20)

½ cup asparagus tips, cooked (20)

½ cup vegetarian baked beans (120)

½ cup broccoli, cooked (25)

½ cup sliced carrots, cooked (25)

½ cup grated carrot (10)

½ cup cauliflower, cooked (25)

1 stalk celery (5)

1 medium ear corn (80)

½ cup sliced cucumber (10)

1 cup green beans, cooked (50)

1 cup mixed salad greens (25)

¼ cup hummus (100)

2 leaves romaine lettuce (0)

½ cup marinara sauce (70)

½ cup chopped red or green bell pepper (15)

2 small (5 oz) red potatoes, baked (100)

1 small (4 oz) sweet potato, baked (95)

1 cup spinach or collards, cooked (20)

2 slices tomato (5)

1 cup tomato-basil soup made with 1% milk (160)

1 can (6 oz.) spicy V-8 (35)

1 cup olive-oil roasted vegetables (130)

1 cup watercress (5)

½ cup sliced zucchini, cooked (25)

WIN THE FAST-FOOD GAME

Even if you want to eat healthy, even if you load your shopping cart with tofu and unidentifiable vegetables, you're probably hard-pressed to log a whole lot of kitchen time. About one-third of us eat fast food on any given day, and about 22 percent eat at convenience stores and fast-food restaurants five or more times a week.

The problem with fast food, of course, is that it's usually *fat* food. When you make the decision to pull into the drive-up lane, you know that you're not going to pull out with a bagful of leafy greens and wholesome grains. You're going to pull out with burgers, fries, a giant Coke—all of the things that are guaranteed to add pounds to your midsection, clog your arteries, and prevent blood from getting to the places where you need it most.

Can you eat fast food and still be healthy? Sure, but only if you're willing to work at it.

We're not going to advise you to give up fast food. You won't do it; we wouldn't do it either. Besides, one of the worst things you can do when you're trying to whip yourself into shape is to give up the foods you love. That's the problem with most diets. They require men to basically take a vow of nutritional chastity, and we all know how well that works. The trick is to allow yourself life's little pleasures—and a steamy bag of crispy fries is obviously among them—without allowing them to cut into your other pleasures, like good sex. Here are a few tricks you'll want to try.

SPLURGE ON FRIES. Just don't do it too often. Ounce for ounce, fries contain more fat than just about any other food. A large order of fries typically has as much fat (and calories) as a quarterpounder. You can't eat them every day if you want to have a prayer of getting in good shape. As a special treat? Sure, go for it.

HOLD THE CHEESE. While you're at it, pass on the bacon. Adding one measly slice of Cheddar to a hamburger vastly increases the fat load. The same goes for the cheese on pizza. While whole-milk mozzarella isn't as fatty as Cheddar, it still delivers about 6 grams of fat per ounce. Then there's the issue of bacon; it's almost pure fat. Go ahead and enjoy burgers and pizza. Have a beer. But hold back on the add-ons. You'll still get most of the eating pleasure, but without the dietary weapons of mass destruction.

DON'T BE FOOLED BY FISH. When you cook it at home, seafood is among the healthiest foods you can eat. But those deep-fried fish fillets from your favorite takeout joint? Almost pure fat. In fact, you'll get just as much calorie-laden fat from most takeout fish fillets as you would if you had the burger.

STEP UP TO THE SALAD BAR. Just about every fast-food joint stocks a lot of salads, vegetables, and the like. Take advantage of them. Even if you just load a small plate, you'll still be filling up stomach space that you'd otherwise pack with burgers and fries. In other words, the salad doesn't have to be a substitute for your main meal, but it will make it easier to eat a little less of the bad stuff.

TRY FAST AND HEALTHY. Not all fast food is fat food. When you're starving and want something quick, a bagel is a good choice. It's high in fiber and practically fat-free, and the complex carbs stay with you, so you won't be eating again in 20 minutes. Other good choices when speed counts: a container of yogurt, those sweet baby carrots, or a handful of nuts. For something more substantial, here are a few things to consider when you're perusing the menu on your lunch break:

▶ Grilled chicken sandwich (get the sauce on the side, and use it sparingly)

▶ Chicken salad with light Italian dressing

▶ Chicken taco salad (hold the sour cream—but get extra guacamole; it's loaded with sex-enhancing vitamin C)

▶ Rotisserie chicken (peel the skin before you eat it)

▶ Chef's salad minus the bacon bits

▶ Veggie or turkey sandwich on whole wheat (get the mayo on the side—or ask for it "lightly spread")

CHAPTER 11

SEX IN A BOTTLE

MAN'S SEARCH FOR THE ELIXIR OF LIFE BEGAN WAY BACK AT THE DAWN OF TIME, WHEN AN OBSERVANT AND NO-DOUBT HUNGRY PROTO-HUMAN DISCOVERED THAT THE HANDFUL OF LEAVES HE CHEWED BEFORE BED MADE HIM FEEL A LITTLE FRISKY. He passed the knowledge on to his mate, who gossiped about it to her girlfriend at the water hole. She, of course, then insisted that *her* man take the magic stuff that could make him go all night. Pretty soon, this tribe of experimenters outpopulated its neighbors, took over the district, and enjoyed the fruits of the first aphrodisiac monopoly.

The rest, as we and the executives at Pfizer (the company that makes Viagra) know, is history—a continuing search for what makes us feel good and last longer.

Yet pharmaceutical shortcuts to better erections are not without risks, side effects, and disappointments. With the exception of men with profound and sometimes serious physical causes of impotence, quick biochemical fixes for sexual dysfunction are rarely as effective as steady transformations through improved physical fitness.

Nonetheless, it makes good sense in some cases to take drugs such as Viagra or to enhance a fitness program with beneficial herbs and essential vitamins and minerals. There's good evidence that some of these products increase energy, boost libido, improve circulation for better erections, and increase the intensity of orgasms.

It's a fact of life: Men don't stay young forever. Erections that you got so easily when you were 20 often become increasingly difficult to achieve or sustain once you reach your 40s and beyond. *"I've definitely noticed that when I date guys who are 5 or 10 years older than me, they seem to have a lower sex drive than I do,"* a 27-year-old Dallas pharmaceutical rep told us.

It doesn't have to be this way. Most men can have the same great sex that they had when they were younger. In fact, it's usually better because of all the experience they picked up along the way. If you're like most men, you don't need a lot of extra help—just a little herbal, nutritional, or chemical nudge to greater levels of sexual pleasure.

ELIXIRS OF LOVE

A woman can have sex whenever she chooses. True, it might take her longer to get ready as she gets older, and she might get less wet than she used to, but she can always pull it off in a pinch. Men, well, have to *stand* to deliver. There's no faking it. After a long and stressful day—and, let's face it, that often means every day—you might not have the physical stamina to achieve a long-lasting erection or the energy for the subsequent lovemaking. This is more likely to occur when you're out of shape, but even the fittest men can ben-

RECREATIONAL MADNESS

Any discussion of recreational drug use has to start with a basic point: It's illegal. Health considerations aside, men who play with them can find themselves trapped in the criminal justice system. It's not a place you want to be.

Now that that's out of the way, let's focus on the sexual issues, starting with marijuana. Some men swear it's an aphrodisiac, and indeed, it can lower inhibitions and make sex more relaxed in some cases. It can also allow users to experience sensations more intensely. Yet the regular use of marijuana decreases testosterone levels and sperm counts, and it may weaken sperm as well. It damages your lungs just as much as cigarettes do. There's no nicotine in marijuana, but it dumps enormous amounts of tar in the lungs. Whoo-ee, doesn't that sound like fun?

The current "it" drug, ecstasy, is a kind of psychedelic-amphetamine hybrid. It's been called the love drug because it makes many users so aroused and energized that they can have sex all night. Fun? Sure, potentially—but the long-term effect on brain cells isn't something you want to mess with.

And there are other drugs that can basically bury your love life.

▶ GHB. Gamma hydroxy butyrate is a chemical compound that's used to strip paint. It first became popular among bodybuilders, who used it after workouts in the belief that it promoted muscle growth. More recently, it's come to be known as one of the date-rape drugs because some users have slipped it into women's drinks to render them unconscious. This stuff is dangerous. Don't touch it.

▶ Amphetamines. Count on impotence or the inability to come. At the same time, they're almost murder on the cardiovascular system. In fact, there probably isn't a body system that can't be seriously damaged by the routine use of amphetamines.

▶ Codeine, Vicodin, OxyContin—the list of abuse drugs goes on and on. It doesn't matter if they're available by prescription. Use them recreationally, and you're going to have trouble, in and out of bed.

efit from a little extra help. Why not take advantage of some "magic" root, berry, fungus, paste, or pill?

Obviously, you don't want to believe every advertisement you read—and the word *magic*, which appears on labels with amazing frequency, should be a full-throated warning that you're about to throw away your money. Manufacturers have been quick to exploit the natural male desire for extra sexual oomph. If you believe that certain herbal concoctions will give you sufficient animal magnetism to lure women away from an absorbing manicure and into your bed, well, there are plenty of charlatans ready to take your money.

As every spammer knows, there's an almost unlimited market for male aphrodisiacs. The path to erection has so many components— the flow of oxygen-rich blood; the stimulation of nerves; and a biochemical flood of hormones, neurotransmitters, and other natural substances—that it's almost inevitable that something will go wrong on occasion. The older you get, the more wrenches fly into the works. Young men often enjoy effortless and frequent erections. It's not so easy when you reach your 30s, 40s, or 50s.

Unfortunately, the marketplace is flooded with products that are ineffective, harmful, or both. On the other hand, there are supplements that have proved their worth over time. A smaller percentage of these supplements, a percentage that's growing all the time, have undergone rigorous scientific testing and proved to be effective.

Most supplements are only marginally regulated by the FDA. Manufacturers aren't required to be very forthcoming, or even particularly truthful, on product labels. If your only experience with supplements is what you read on the boxes or bottles, you'll find yourself spending serious money on products that probably don't work. That said, you don't have to do a dissertation's worth of research to discover that some active ingredients in herbs and other supplements *do* make a difference. The same is true of some vitamins and minerals. When these products are incorporated into an overall healthy lifestyle and used as part of a well-rounded fitness program, they really can make a difference.

Most supplements, incidentally, don't deliver the same "stand back!" experience as prescription drugs. (And some prescription drugs, as you'll see, might not live up to their overhyped reputations.) Their full effects might not be evident for weeks or even months. A good rule of thumb is to give a supplement (with the possible exception of standard vitamins and minerals) 6 weeks to work. If you haven't noticed anything by then, it's probably safe to scratch it off as a dud.

THE PILL THAT MAKES YOU HARDER

Viagra, the little blue pill that some devotees call vitamin V, was the first really important gift from modern science to men with erection problems. The active ingredient, sildenafil citrate, blocks an enzyme and allows a chemical called cyclic GMP to relax the smooth muscles in your penis. In other words, it causes blood vessels to relax and engorge with blood. More blood is the key to getting hard.

That's not the whole story, of course. Viagra is not an aphrodisiac. You don't get an instant erection when you take it. It doesn't increase your libido, your staying power, or your normal frequency of erections. All it does is fine-tune your machinery so that you can get an erection at the appropriate time. You still have to do your part by doing or watching the kinds of things that get you excited.

Even if your only Internet experience is sending e-mails and taking an occasional look at the Victoria's Secret Web site, you probably know that Viagra is readily available from online merchants. The prices aren't necessarily better than what you'd pay at a regular pharmacy, but many men appreciate the anonymity of the transactions. You don't have to go through the embarrassment of talking with your doctor. All you have to do on most of these sites is fill out a cursory medical history and hand over your credit card number.

The problem with this approach, of course, is that you aren't getting any real medical supervision—and despite what you may have heard, Viagra isn't 100 percent safe for everyone, and for a minority of men, it poses significant risks. If you have heart problems and are taking drugs such as nitroglycerine, for example, Viagra could kill you. There's also the risk that it could worsen underlying conditions you don't even know you have. Viagra is no different in this sense from any other prescription drug. You really need to see a doctor

NOT SO FAST—AND NOT SO HARD

One of nature's ironies is that teenagers, who have far more interest in sex than opportunities for getting it, constantly get erections at inopportune times. Older men who can count on sex, on the other hand, are often resigned to waiting impatiently, teeth gnashing, for the eventual appearance of "wood."

True, you don't have to walk around with a magazine in your pocket for emergency concealment purposes. On the other hand, it would be nice to be ready for sex without having to wait for it—and without having to apologize to the occasional, less-than-gentle partner who regards it as a personal affront if you aren't instantly hard in her presence.

You'll just have to live with it. It's normal for men ages 30 and older to take more time than they once did to get an erection. In addition, just thinking sexy thoughts is unlikely to have the same effect that it used to. As men age, they need more direct physical stimulation to get hard and stay hard.

There is an upside to all of this. Older men are less likely than the young guys to be burdened with hair triggers, which means they can take their time and enjoy sex more.

before taking it. Oh, and since so many of these sites are unregulated, the little blue pills you receive might not even contain the active ingredient. Worse, they might contain harmful substances.

This caveat aside, Viagra really is a remarkable drug. About 80 percent of men who take it report significant improvement in their ability to get erections—and the erections are usually harder than they were before. If you're planning to try Viagra, here are a few points to keep in mind.

CUT AND SAVE. Viagra comes in three doses: 25-, 50-, and 100-milligram tablets. Your doctor will probably start you on the lower dose—but you should still ask for the 100-milligram tablets. Viagra is expensive, upward of $10 a pill in most cases, and the price for all doses is roughly the same. The cheapest way to use it is to get a prescription for the 100-milligram pills, then cut them into halves or quarters, following your doctor's advice.

The good folks at Pfizer haven't bothered to score the pills, so they don't break easily. You might want to pick up a pill splitter at a pharmacy. They cost only a few bucks and make it easy to cut 100-milligram pills down to size.

TAKE IT AN HOUR BEFORE YOU NEED IT. Some men report getting erections within half an hour after taking Viagra. An hour is about right for most men, and there's a 4- to 5-hour window of opportunity before the effects wear off. Viagra works more quickly when there's not a lot of food in your stomach—so don't expect instant results if you and your date have just polished off a couple of filet mignons. Also, don't take Viagra more than once a day, and don't exceed a daily dose of 100 milligrams.

MONITOR YOUR PROGRESS. Recent studies show that about 20 percent of men who take Viagra stop responding to the standard dose after about 2 years. Increasing the dose will usually restore its effectiveness, but not always. Doctors aren't sure at this point if men simply build up a tolerance to the drug, or if the reduction in effectiveness is due to a worsening of the underlying problems, such as nerve or blood vessel damage, that caused the erection problems in the first place. In any event, let your doctor know if you're not responding. There are other drugs available, and undoubtedly, there will be more in the coming years.

NOT-SO-SEXY STEROIDS

Don't confuse the steroids that doctors sometimes give to men who have low libido, impotence, or other sexual problems with the steroids that practically spill off the shelves in some locker rooms. They're entirely different beasts.

You naturally manufacture some steroids in the adrenal glands or testicles. You need natural steroids such as testosterone to function sexually. The drugs used by some athletes, on the other hand, are anabolic steroids. They're manufactured in laboratories and consumed by people who are apparently more interested in growing muscles the size of an Angus bull's than taking care of their health.

It's not surprising that these drugs are popular among athletes seeking a competitive edge. Besides producing that unmistakably beefy appearance, anabolic steroids decrease the recovery time required following workouts or mild injuries. Men who take them are able to work out harder and gain more endurance at the same time.

A lot of men swear they're good for sex as well. Sorry, not true. Some men who take steroids have an obvious increase in breast size and a decrease in the size of their testicles—not exactly the kinds of changes your significant other is likely to welcome. Sperm counts drop in men who take steroids. Erections? History, for the most part; impotence is a common side effect. Then there are the really serious side effects, such as an increased risk of prostate cancer.

BE ALERT TO SIDE EFFECTS. They're usually minor, but they can be unsettling if you don't expect them. Men who take Viagra often experience some nasal congestion and facial flushing. Others have stomach upset, headaches, or dizziness. Perhaps the strangest side effect is the blue haze that some men report. It can last a few minutes or several hours, and this, along with Viagra's blue color, has earned it the street nickname "blues." Research has shown that the blue haze affects about 3 percent of men who take Viagra.

OTHER ERECTION DRUGS

We've been talking about Viagra in detail because it was the first popular oral drug for erection problems and because it's the drug that most men are familiar with. In the past few years, however, two new drugs with similar effects, Cialis (tadalafil) and Levitra (vardenafil), have been approved by the FDA. They're very expensive at this point, but the prices will undoubtedly drop eventually.

So far, doctors haven't done head-to-head comparisons of the three drugs. No one can say at this point which one is best for most men. Viagra and Levitra have very similar effects and side effects. Cialis is a little different because it starts working in about half the time, and its effects last 24 to 36 hours—which means you don't have to make a mental note to take it an hour before having sex. You might take it on a Friday night, for example, and it could continue working through much of the weekend.

HORMONES FOR MEN

Hormone therapy (HT) for men is a somewhat controversial treatment that falls in the gray area between medical necessity and fad treatment. Its use, and its burgeoning popularity, is often linked to the relatively new concept of andropause, or male menopause.

Researchers have known for a long time that a man's level of testosterone, the male hormone that fuels libido and erections, steadily declines with age. Most endocrinologists, doctors who specialize in the complex interplay of the body's hormones, believe that the drop in testosterone is pretty insignificant, at least in terms of sexual performance. But some doctors, primarily those who specialize in a relatively new field known as anti-aging medicine, believe that flagging levels of testosterone are responsible for many of the symptoms of male malaise—not only declines in libido and the firmness of erections but also low energy, depression, and memory loss. A study of 890 older men by researchers from the Baltimore Longitudinal Study on Aging found that 20 percent of subjects in their 60s had lower than normal testosterone levels, 30 percent in their 70s had levels below normal, and half of men in their 80s were testosterone deficient.

There is some evidence that synthetic forms of testosterone, such as Andryl 200, Delatestryl, Depo-Testosterone, and Virilon IM, may improve erections in some men, especially when combined with drugs such as Viagra. And there's no question that men who are truly deficient in testosterone require treatment with HT.

But the key question, and one that can't be answered with any certainty yet, is whether HT can jump-start libido (or energy, or anything else) in otherwise healthy men. For now, most mainstream doctors restrict the use of this approach to men who have undergone lab tests and been found to have hormone deficiencies or imbalances. It's not given routinely, especially because testosterone treatments can fuel the growth of prostate and other cancers.

Whatever you do, don't take these drugs without medical supervision. The doses have to be calibrated with a lot of precision, and the drugs, when used inappropriately or taken by men with other health problems, can increase the risk of stroke, heart attack, or other serious health threats.

VITAMINS AND MINERALS

If your idea of a green vegetable is a martini olive, and you get most of your carbs from doughnuts and pretzels, your sex life may be paying the price.

Yes, you need optimal levels of vitamins and minerals to protect your heart, build muscle, and strengthen bones. And yes, your risk of getting sick is a lot higher if you don't eat a fundamentally nutritious diet, preferably one that's bolstered with a daily multivitamin/mineral supplement. But forget all that and focus on what's *really* important: You need a few key nutrients to maintain or improve sex drive as well as performance.

In an ideal world, we'd all eat the way nutritionists tell us to: five or more daily servings of fruits and vegetables, plenty of legumes and whole grains, minimal amounts of fat, and so on. But who has time to think about all that, especially when you're leaving the office at 7 o'clock, and your stomach essentially drags you to the nearest drive-thru lane? Even if you make a conscientious effort to eat well, your intake of key nutrients is probably on the low side, if only because so many of the foods we eat have been stripped of their natural nutritional payloads. The cells in your body, including those that make up your sexual machinery, pay the price by working at less than peak capacity.

Get in the habit of taking a multivitamin/mineral supplement. It won't miraculously boost your endurance or improve your ability to have erections, but it can give you a little edge. Obviously, every man needs a different mix of nutrients, depending on his diet and lifestyle. If you really want to do it right, see a doctor who special-

HOW MUCH IS ENOUGH?

Unless you have a doctorate in nutrition, it's a real bear keeping track of all the assorted vitamins and minerals that you need for sexual health. The basic rule when supplementing is to take up to the recommended Daily Values (DVs). It's best to first check with a doctor or qualified practitioner if you're thinking of taking higher amounts. The values are set by the FDA and meet the basic nutritional needs for most men.

VITAMINS	100% DAILY VALUE
A	5,000 international units (IU)
B_6	2 milligrams (mg)
B_{12}	6 micrograms (mcg)
C	60 mg
D	400 IU
E	30 IU
Folic Acid	400 mcg
K	80 mcg
Niacin (vitamin B_3)	20 mg
Riboflavin (vitamin B_2)	1.7 mg
Thiamin (vitamin B_1)	1.5 mg

MINERALS	100% DAILY VALUE
Calcium	1,000 mg
Chloride	3,400 mg
Chromium	120 mcg
Copper	2 mg
Iodine	150 mcg
Iron	18 mg
Magnesium	400 mg
Phosphorus	1,000 mg
Potassium	3,500 mg
Selenium	70 mcg
Zinc	15 mg

izes in nutritional health to find out where you need the most help. In most cases, the nutrients below, starting with the ones men need most, are the ones that have been shown to make the biggest difference.

GET HARDER WITH ZINC. It's probably the most important mineral for men because it's used by the body for the synthesis of testosterone. Low zinc potentially means low testosterone—which means you won't be frying any eggs on your libido until you turn things around. Men who don't get enough zinc are also likely to have uncomfortable brushes with impotence. One study at the Grand Forks Human Nutrition Research Center in North Dakota found that 11 young men who were fed low-, medium-, and high-zinc diets had significantly lower levels of testosterone and lower semen volumes after eating the diet lowest in zinc for 35 days.

Your body does more with zinc than manufacture testosterone. The mineral also helps maintain an adequate sperm count and makes the penis healthier. A study by Singapore researchers compared zinc levels in the semen of 107 infertile and 103 fertile men. Those who were infertile had an average zinc level of 184 milligrams per liter compared with an average of 275 in the fertile men. The men with lower zinc levels also had lower sperm quality and motility. Zinc is also believed to sharpen your senses, especially your sense of taste and smell—and you know how important those are as part of satisfying sexual encounters.

If you smoke or drink a lot of alcohol or coffee, incidentally, you'll really burn through the zinc. Make an effort to eat plenty of zinc-rich foods, such as tuna, oysters, oats, peas, and lentils. It's also a good idea to take a multi supplement that contains zinc, especially if your lifestyle habits aren't exactly on the saintly side.

TAKE THE "SEX VITAMIN." Vitamin E is one nutrient that deserves its racy reputation. It plays a key role in shipping blood to tissues throughout the body, including the penis. You need that blood for good erections. In addition, vitamin E is among the most potent antioxidants. It blocks the harmful molecules in the body that damage blood vessel walls and increase buildups of plaque, the fatty stuff that's a common cause of soft (or nonexistent) erections. Men who have diabetes are especially prone to damaged blood vessel walls, which is one reason why more than half of all men with diabetes are impotent. A study of men with and without diabetes found that those who were impotent had significantly lower vitamin E levels compared with those who did not have erectile dysfunction.

Check with your doctor first, but taking vitamin E with aspirin can significantly reduce your risk of heart disease—and the antioxidant-and-blood-thinner combination can reduce the blood-blocking arterial deposits that inhibit erections.

Vitamin E is found mainly in plant oils, along with salmon, eggs, almonds, and leafy vegetables such as spinach. It's hard to get enough from food alone, however. Of all the nutritional supplements, this is the one that your doctor is most likely to recommend. Plan on taking 400 IU daily. This is higher than the Daily Value, so check with your doctor before taking that much.

GET ENOUGH POTASSIUM. It balances acidity in the glands and aids in the creation of testosterone. You also need potassium for healthy nerves and muscles; men who are low in this mineral may experience diminished sexual responsiveness and coordination.

Plus, potassium helps regulate blood pressure, and a study of 776 men in the Massachusetts Male Aging Study found that having high blood pressure doubled a man's risk of developing erectile dysfunction over 10 years. Another study of 54 people taking high blood pressure medication found that 81 percent of those who ate a potassium-rich diet for a year were able to cut their drug dosages significantly.

It doesn't hurt to take a daily supplement that contains potassium, but it's pretty easy to get enough as long as you eat lean meats and nuts, along with whole grains and fruits and vegetables.

PUMP SOME IRON. Low energy in the sack? You might be low in iron, the mineral that allows red blood cells to carry oxygen to tissues in the penis and elsewhere in the body. You won't have any trouble getting enough iron as long as you eat lean meat, eggs, raisins, bananas, and green vegetables.

STRENGTHEN SPERM WITH C. If you're thinking about starting a family, now's the time to slug down some OJ. Vitamin C increases sperm count and motility, the ability of the little squigglers to get more closely acquainted with that alluring egg. A study of 13 infertile men who were given 1,000 milligrams of vitamin C twice a day for 2 months found that the men's sperm counts more than doubled, and sperm motility improved significantly.

Vitamin C improves the absorption of iron and aids in the production of the hormones that minimize stress—essential if you're hoping to have a good time when the lights go down. In one study, lab rats were confined an hour a day to increase their stress hormones. When they were fed the human equivalent of a few grams of vitamin C daily for 3 weeks, their stress hormone levels fell.

Nearly every multivitamin contains adequate amounts of vitamin C. You'll get even more if you eat citrus fruits, tomatoes, peppers, onions, and other fruits and vegetables.

SIMPLIFY WITH A COMPLEX. There are 11 different B vitamins, and you can easily drive yourself crazy figuring out how much of each you need. An easier approach is to take a B-complex supplement that includes all of these important nutrients. You need B vitamins for healthy muscles and nerves and to enhance fertility, boost circulation and the production of red blood cells, and increase energy and libido. Foods rich in B vitamins include fish, brewer's yeast, legumes, eggs, and brown rice and other whole grains.

CRANK UP THE CALCIUM. You already know that you need calcium for strong bones. What you may not know is that this common mineral, one of the electrolytes, is essential for the transmission of nerve signals—signals that allow the brain to efficiently communicate with the penis. Been trying some unusual positions lately? Definitely make sure you get enough calcium. Muscles need it to contract, and low levels can leave you gasping with painful, sex-stopping cramps.

Calcium also helps to keep both your blood pressure and your weight in check, and high blood pressure and obesity raise your risk of having erection problems. A survey conducted by the Harvard School of Public Health looked at the profiles of nearly 2,000 men over age 50. Those with erectile dysfunction were more likely to have high blood pressure and be overweight. In fact, men with 42-inch waistlines were nearly twice as likely to have erection problems as men whose waists measured 32 inches.

A few glasses of milk or fortified juice daily will provide all the calcium you need. Other calcium-rich foods include yogurt, most breakfast cereals, and sardines (with the bones).

IMPROVE VIGOR WITH VITAMIN A. Your body needs this nutrient to utilize the testosterone that's already present. It also strengthens testicular tissue, maintains healthy sperm levels, and inhibits the accumulation of artery-clogging gunk. You'll get plenty if you take a daily multivitamin or eat foods such as liver; eggs; and yellow and green vegetables, such as carrots, sweet potatoes, and spinach.

HERBS AND SUPPLEMENTS

The modern pharmaceutical industry has been lobbying politicians for decades to do everything but take herbal medicines off pharmacy and health-food store shelves. You can hardly blame them. After all, all of those leaves, roots, and twigs grow free for the picking, so to speak. They're certainly a fraction of the cost of high-tech drugs. Doctors, not the most liberal bunch in town, love to talk about the inadequate testing of herbal remedies as well as the so-called dangers—though their own medical journals report that only a handful of people are harmed by herbs each year, while prescription and over-the-counter drugs are among the leading causes of injury and death in the United States.

▼

The ancient Aztecs believed that avocados conferred uncontrollable sexual desire. Even being in proximity to one of these testicle-shaped fruits was thought to get libido raging—which is why young women, especially virgins, were required to keep a cautious distance.

▲

It's true that most herbal remedies haven't been rigorously studied, but this has more to do with money than anything else. No pharmaceutical company worth its stockholders will spend millions of dollars studying natural plant compounds that can't be patented—and will never generate the gargantuan profits the industry is accustomed to. Even doctors who specialize in alternative medicine wish there were more studies to conclusively show which herbs work best, what the safest doses are, and which patients are most likely to benefit. Until those studies are done, herbal medicine will continue to represent more of a process of trial and error than one of predictable results.

Still, recent studies have shown that many herbs do appear to live up to their age-old reputations. Indeed, the pharmaceutical industry spends a fortune sending scientists around the globe to collect and analyze plants. They have no intention of actually marketing herbs in their natural forms, of course. Instead, they use plant molecules as basic templates to create "unique" molecules that can bring astronomical profits.

All those drugs in your medicine cabinet? A least a quarter of them contain active ingredients that are similar or identical to those found in plants. The herb St. John's wort, for example, has been shown in clinical studies to be as effective for mild to moderate depression as the Prozac-like drugs. You might need insulin to control diabetes, but there's good evidence that a clove of garlic daily can naturally lower blood sugar. And because the active ingredients in these and other herbs are much less concentrated than drugs, they enter the body more slowly and are less likely to cause miserable side effects.

We've been talking about herbs, but many of the same arguments apply to nonherbal supplements as well. Doctors don't trust them; scientists have just begun to study them; and millions of men, who tend to trust their own experiences at least as much as the opinions of medical talking heads, are willing to give them a try.

Obviously, there are plenty of herbs and supplements that won't do a thing for your love life, no matter what the manufacturers say. Others really work, though not as dramatically as some men expect. Herbs and supplements aren't like drugs. You often have to take them for a long time before noticing any appreciable benefits—and those benefits are likely to be pretty subtle. Don't take these products indefinitely if you don't notice a difference, say, within a month or two. Cut your losses and move on.

One final word before we look at some of the specific products that can make a real difference in your sexual health. Always take the amount listed on the label. More is unlikely to be helpful and may increase the risk of side effects. Also, some herbs and supplements block or increase the effects of prescription drugs. Do let your doctor know what you're taking if you're receiving medical treatment for other conditions, and don't mess around with products if you have any doubt about their effectiveness or safety.

We've listed the following herbs and supplements in order of their potential to benefit you—especially your potential for harder, better, longer sex.

IMPROVE ERECTIONS WITH YOHIMBINE. An herb often sold in supplement form, yohimbine once had the stamp of approval of the FDA and was sold by prescription as a treatment for impotence. The FDA has since reversed itself, but there's good evidence that yohimbine really does help, mainly by dilating blood vessels and increasing bloodflow to the penis. Two different analyses in the late 1990s that reviewed a combined 23 studies showed that yohimbine is an effective treatment for erection problems. But a 1995 FDA analysis of 26 over-the-counter products found that many didn't contain enough yohimbine to really help. Still, those who try it say they notice a difference.

"I've taken yohimbine, and it slightly improved my ability to maintain an erection and regain it after intercourse," a 45-year-old certified public accountant told us.

Yohimbine has effects similar to those of adrenaline, one of the "fight or flight" hormones. It can potentially elevate heart rate as well as blood pressure. If you already have high blood pressure or heart problems, definitely don't take it without your doctor's okay.

GAIN ENERGY WITH GINSENG. The root has been used as a general tonic throughout Asia for centuries. Herbalists claim that it improves physical and mental health and enhances athletic and sexual performance. There does seem to be something to it. A study reported in *Drugs in Experimental and Clinical Research* found that people who took a daily multivitamin supplement along with ginseng felt better overall than those who only took the vitamin.

Like yohimbine, ginseng may improve bloodflow to the penis by dilating blood vessels. It also appears to improve nerve function, essential for healthy erections. Two placebo-controlled studies by Korean researchers found ginseng helped men with erection problems.

Don't take ginseng if you have high blood pressure or hypoglycemia. Because it's sold in so many forms—whole root, powder, liquid extract, capsules, and so on—it's a challenge to figure out which one to use. As a rule of thumb, look for the word *Panax* on the label, which means that the herb is American or Asian in origin. Siberian ginseng, found in some products, has not been as well studied. It's also important to buy a standardized formula containing 15 percent ginsenosides; that means the manufacturers have tested the product to ensure that there are sufficient quantities of the active ingredient. Doctors recommend starting with 1 to 2 grams a day.

GET EXCITED BY MUIRA PUAMA. When 262 men took 1 to 1.5 grams of muira puama extract (nicknamed potency wood) daily for 2 weeks, 51 percent reported better erections, and 62 percent said it helped their libidos.

HELP YOUR GENITALS BREATHE. It sounds strange, but tissues throughout your body need oxygen to function at full capacity. The herb damiana is particularly good because it promotes the flow of oxygen to the penis and testicles. It's a common ingredient in male potency tonics and has been used for centuries as an aphrodisiac. It's doubtful that it really adds fuel to your sexual fire, but it does appear to improve overall sexual health and performance. One study in rats showed that the herb improved sexual performance in previously "sluggish" animals.

Because damiana interferes with the body's absorption of iron, however, you don't want to take more than the amount listed on the label. Eat plenty of iron-rich foods to counteract its iron-draining effects. Also, be warned that some men who take damiana experience nausea or digestive upset. Definitely stop taking it if you experience these or other side effects.

GET COOKING WITH CINNAMON. Yep, this kitchen herb can jump-start your libido. Studies have shown, in fact, that men who simply inhale the aroma of cinnamon have increases in sexual desire. Cinnamon also appears to enhance circulation and improve overall vitality. Tests by researchers at the Smell and Taste Treatment and Research Foundation in Chicago found that the aroma of cinnamon was the only scent among dozens that brought on erections in the participants.

WAKE UP DESIRE WITH GINKGO. It's among the most popular herbal remedies, one of the safest—and one of the best for better sex. One study found that people taking antidepressants, which are notorious for depressing libido, had a jump in sexual desire when they added ginkgo to the mix. In an often-cited 1989 German study, ginkgo was found to reverse impotence. Sixty men with erection problems caused by impaired bloodflow to the penis took ginkgo daily for a year, and half of them regained the ability to have erections after 6 months. And a small study presented at a national urology conference in 1998 found that overnight erections were slightly more rigid in men who took ginkgo than in men who took a placebo.

The herb is considered safe in doses up to 240 milligrams a day, but doctors usually suggest starting at 80 milligrams. One caution: The combination of ginkgo and aspirin has caused complications in a few patients, so check with your doc if you take aspirin regularly.

TRY *AVENA SATIVA*. This green oat straw has been a staple of sex formulas because it may help alleviate sexual problems (especially low libido) by raising testosterone levels. In one study, 20 men who took 300 milligrams a day of green oat extract experienced a 54 percent increase in frequency of sexual activity.

TAKE SAW PALMETTO. But only if you have an enlarged prostate, which could cause sexual problems by interfering with the

nerves and blood vessels that feed your penis. Relieving the condition may help you attain erections. Studies of men with enlarged
prostates have found that saw palmetto significantly relieved their
symptoms. Look for extracts that are standardized to contain 85
percent fatty acids.

If you have an enlarged prostate, most doctors suggest taking 320
milligrams a day. If you don't, taking saw palmetto may actually
worsen your sexual performance because it reduces the production
of testosterone.

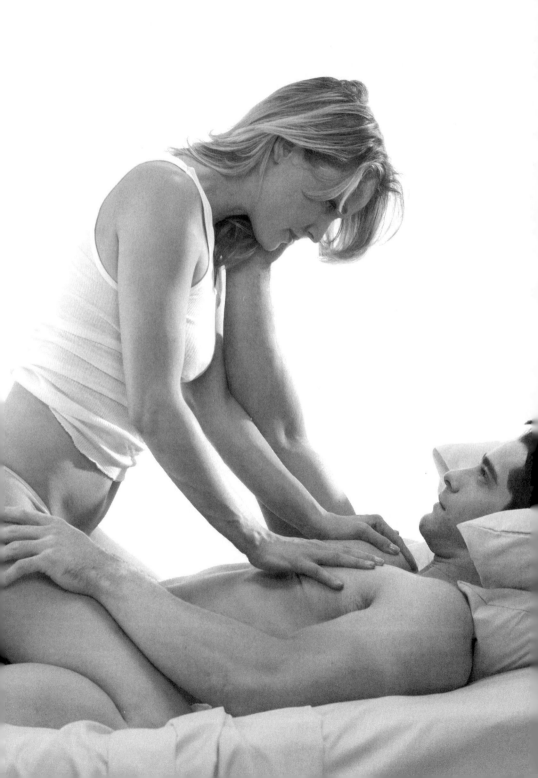

PART 5

TROUBLE
IN PARADISE

CHAPTER 12

MIND MATTERS

**MEN WHO TALK ABOUT THEIR EROGENOUS ZONES USU-
ALLY GRIN AND POINT BELOW THE BELT, AS THOUGH A
LITTLE STIMULATION *THERE* IS ALL THEY NEED TO GET
HOT.** Forget for a moment that various parts of our anatomy are
exquisitely sensitive. Forget, too, that most of us need a variety of
stimuli, such as a sexy kiss, a lick of the nipples, or a hard bite on
the neck, to get really aroused. The *real* sex organ, the one that controls all of your pleasures and desires, is the one on top of your
neck. The brain is the ultimate source of sexual joy. It's also, for a
lot of men, the source of sexual disappointment.

How many times have you been thinking about sex, or maybe
even having it, when you suddenly realize that you're not all there?
Your body might be willing, but your mind is miles away. Maybe
you argued with your partner, and you're still a little stressed. Or
your head's filled with images of overdue credit card bills. Or you
haven't been working out and are self-conscious about the way you
look. Like it or not, sex is intertwined with the rest of your life.

When you're stressed, tired, or depressed, your libido—and erections—will probably pack their bags for an extended vacation.

Psychologists who specialize in male sexual dysfunction say that mental barriers are among the greatest obstacles to good sex. The sexiest video, the most sensual massage, the most imaginative and uninhibited foreplay won't do much when your brain is saying "Nah." We all have times in our lives when baggage from the past and pressure in the present keep intruding in the bedroom. It might not happen all the time or even very often, but a few nights of sexual disappointment will convince you that you're damn tired of the extra company.

You might decide to enlist the advice of a pro to help you sort out your issues, sexual and otherwise. It's unlikely, though, that you need heavy-duty counseling (though a few sessions can always help). You probably need to just tweak your thinking to get a better grip on how you approach your life, in and out of the bedroom.

WHEN YOUR BODY MESSES WITH YOUR MIND

Women are always talking about their weight, their hair, how much they hate their bodies. It's true that our looks-conscious culture gnaws away at women's self-esteem long before they reach middle school. It's always mind-boggling to read stories about the world's most beautiful women and discover that these goddesses find their bodies to be perfectly loathsome.

For a long time, experts who studied the effects of body image on psychological health focused mainly on women. It's only in the past few years that they've come to understand that men have many of the same issues. The images in our heads of idealized male physiques, and the way the world responds to them (while ignoring us mere mortals), conspire to make us view ourselves in less than positive ways.

The way you see yourself powerfully affects, for good or bad, your sexual confidence. Unfortunately, the messages we get from the earliest ages aren't always the ones that build us up. It's painful to watch some overbearing dad come down hard when his son doesn't throw a perfect spiral pass or handle an ax with the skill of Paul Bunyan. Imagine growing up and knowing that your dad, the most important man in your life, is disappointed when you aren't manly enough. Memories like this last a lifetime.

Then there's the joy of the schoolyard, the only place on Earth that's crueler than a Soviet-era gulag. Kids in packs are merciless, and few boys escape the endless taunts: "Lard-ass." "Pencil-neck." "Loser."

Once a man becomes an adult, he's beset with media images that make it very clear that the average guy with an average body is about as sexy as an old sock. Despite evidence to the contrary, these images make it seem as though women lust for only hunks with hot bodies. Those actors and models are viewed as icons of manliness—never mind that those "ideal" features were created with a surgeon's knife or the sweep of an airbrush.

Once a man internalizes the message that he somehow doesn't measure up, his ability to enjoy sex, or even have it at all, starts to head south. You've probably seen guys who walk all hunched up, as though they're instinctively trying to protect themselves. They're so self-conscious that they barely move their bodies. Multiply that by years, and it's no

▼

You need to be healthy to have good sex—but frequent sex can also make you healthy. Animal species that behave promiscuously tend to have higher levels of white blood cells and greater resistance to infection. In human studies, those who have sex twice weekly have higher levels of immunoglobulin A, a disease-fighting antibody. They're also half as likely to have a heart attack or stroke.

▲

wonder that their muscles get weak and stiff. They become almost detached from their own bodies, ignoring their wants and needs or actually abusing them. At the same time, they don't think highly enough of themselves to invest money in sharp-looking clothes, so they really do become less attractive to others.

It's an ugly cycle, one that traps all of us to one degree or another. The only way to achieve true sexual happiness is to somehow get off that self-destructive treadmill.

Here's what you can expect. When you improve your body, you shape up mentally as well. There's nothing like feeling strong and energized to boost your self-image, self-control, and sexual confidence. Study after study has shown that men who exercise regularly are less likely to be depressed and more likely to do the kinds of things that make them feel strong and sexy. There are all sorts of reasons for this. Here are a few examples.

▶ Exercise improves strength, stamina, and cardiovascular conditioning, key components for energetic, creative sex. At the same time, exercise can vastly improve libido. Men with a strong appetite for sex are usually the ones who feel strong physically. A landmark study by researchers at the University of California in San Diego looked at 78 previously sedentary men who followed a moderate aerobic regimen four times a week. After 9 months, the men reported that their frequency of sexual intercourse jumped an average of 30 percent, with 26 percent more orgasms. They also reported increased frequency of masturbation.

▶ Exercise, even if it's nothing more vigorous than swimming a few laps or walking for half an hour, stimulates the release of endorphins and adrenaline, brain chemicals that play key roles in the chemistry of sexual arousal. One Italian study of 2,400 men revealed that those with erectile dysfunction were significantly less likely to be physically active.

▶ Lifting weights, especially when you concentrate on the big muscles in the arms, chest, shoulders, and back, has been shown to increase confidence and self-esteem. If you do it long enough, you'll notice impressive changes in your body that make you feel sexier. You'll *look* sexier too. Plus, weight training can boost your body's natural production of testosterone, which in turn can boost your sex drive.

▶ Combining weight workouts with aerobic workouts will literally flood your body with endorphins while reducing levels of stress hormones—chemical downers that are like death to good sex. In a 1999 study reported in the *Canadian Journal of Applied Physiology*, resting levels of the stress hormone cortisol decreased 17 percent over 20 weeks of weight training. At the same time, exercise helps you sleep better. Men who wake up fresh have more energy and confidence—two qualities that act almost like aphrodisiacs, not only for you but for your partner as well.

Convinced? You should be. Researchers have found that men who embark on an exercise program start feeling better about themselves almost as soon as they start—long before any obvious physical changes take hold. There's something about being physically active that makes you a storehouse of animal energy. In fact, you'll start to feel like the animal you are—a predator, a hunter, a man who's at his best when he's sleek, supple, and strong.

SEXY SHUT-EYE

Without air, you're pretty much a goner in 3 minutes. A man deprived of water for just 3 days is likewise toast. Then there's heat. Jump off the deck of a transatlantic ocean liner, and you'll live less than an hour in the 45-degree swells.

Air, water, heat: the human big three. Next on the list, even before food, comes sleep. You'll start to seriously hallucinate within 72 hours if you don't sleep. Loopy disorientation usually sets in long before then.

Small wonder, then, that men with insomnia are so tired—or disoriented—that they can hardly muster the desire or the ability to

TAKE THE STRESS TEST

Stress is such an integral part of modern life that it's not always easy to tell what's normal and what's not. After all, what would seem to be iron-clad proof of stress in one man—say, screaming at a referee's idiotic call—would be entirely normal, if boorish, in another.

If you experience one or more of the following on a regular basis, consider it a warning flare that your life, and sooner or later your sex life, is on the wrong track.

Messed-up eating. You're either gorging on food or not eating enough. Any long-term change in your normal appetite can be caused by stress as well as depression.

Junk-food frenzies. There's some evidence that men unconsciously attempt to self-treat stress and depression by dumping sugar and carbs into the bloodstream. These foods can elevate levels of body chemicals that make you feel better, at least temporarily. The good feelings are invariably followed by a crash, of course, which increases stress over time.

Fatigue. If you're tired all the time or aren't sleeping well, you can bet that your stress levels are rising.

Temper, temper. Everyone gets mad sometimes. Guys who are stressed *always* seem to be on the edge of volcanic venting.

Restlessness. If you've always been a cool sort of dude, but lately you've been jiggling your legs, playing with change in your pocket, or popping up from your desk every 5 minutes, take a look at the pressures in your life. They might be getting out of hand.

have sex. It makes sense. Sex, though it doesn't always seem like it at the time, is an optional activity; you won't die without it. But your body does have to maintain itself. Sleep is the time when essential chemicals are restored and damaged cells repaired. Without sleep, your brain simply can't function. Given a choice between sex and restorative sleep, your body will choose sleep every time. And this obstacle affects the sex lives of more men than you might imagine. A poll by the National Sleep Foundation found that nearly one-quarter of American adults aren't getting enough sleep.

Sex is a great cure for sleepless nights, of course. Your tense body and overwrought mind will start to unwind when you're in contact with a loving human touch. But if you don't get enough sleep in the first place, you'll probably be too tired to have sex, whether or not someone's in bed with you. Then there's the issue of what's giving you sleepless nights in the first place. For most men, it's stress. A recent study of 59 adults by researchers at the University of Pittsburgh found that stress caused heart-rate changes that altered the nervous system's natural sleep cycle, depriving stressed participants of much-needed deep sleep.

Doctors in sleep clinics see a lot of men who can't get erections or who report low libidos. They say that the endless cycle of insomnia followed by stress followed by sexual *distress* can put you totally out of commission. Insomnia, as well as the sleep disorder called sleep apnea, lowers testosterone levels, reduces sex drive, and makes you, to use the clinical term, wacky. You can certainly drug yourself to sleep, but even the most benign sleeping pills can hamper your libido even more.

To save your sleep *and* have better sex, here's what doctors advise.

FOLLOW THE 3-HOUR RULE. Plan to do a 30-minute aerobic workout within 3 hours before hitting the sheets. Actually, any exercise during the day will help you sleep, but this 3-hour window is optimal for good shut-eye. Don't put off your workout until the last minute, however. Men who exercise in the last hour before bed may get too wound up to fall asleep right away.

SLEEP BY THE CLOCK. Yes, life is unpredictable, and it's easy to get caught up in a cycle of erratic sleep times—staying up until midnight on weekends, crashing at 9 P.M. on Sundays, and so on. You have to train your body to start winding down at the end of the day, and the best way to do it is to go to bed and get up at roughly the same times every day.

NIX THE NAPS. There will obviously be times when you're so wasted during the day that your only recourse is to lie on the couch and pass out for half an hour. That's fine on occasion, but you don't want to get into the habit of having daytime snoozes. It's obvious that men who nap during the day are going to have more trouble falling asleep at night.

If nothing else, keep your naps to less than 30 minutes. Longer than that will plunge you into deep, slow-wave sleep and cut into your nighttime z's.

GET UP IF YOU HAVE TO. Even though you want to keep regular sleep hours, don't try to force yourself to sleep if it isn't happening. Give yourself about 20 minutes to fall asleep. If you're not out by then, get out of bed for awhile and do something else. Sit in the living room and have a cup of chamomile tea, nature's equivalent of sleeping pills. Watch some TV. Do some dishes. Don't go back to bed until the yawns start taking over.

SAVE THE BEDROOM FOR SLEEP. Okay, you can make an exception for sex or reading the latest Tom Clancy novel. But that's it. Don't use your bedroom as a temporary office. Don't spread your

> ▼
> **Headache researchers have found that sex is an almost instant cure for skull-pounders, probably because it improves brain circulation—and because having an orgasm triggers the release of pain-blocking endorphins. The same brain chemicals can temporarily ease mild depression as well.**
> ▲

bills all over the bed at the end of the month. The more stressful activities you bring into the bedroom, the more stress you put into your head every time you walk in the door. You want your brain to say, "Hey, I'm in the bedroom; must be time to wind down."

RELAX AND DE-STRESS

We've got it pretty good in this country—but nothing in life is free. We pay quite a price for a life awash in cell phones, food processors, and satellite TVs. For starters, you have to work to pay for all that stuff. Men today spend a lot more hours securing the so-called basics than their cave-dwelling ancestors ever dreamed of. Anthropologists estimate that our primitive forebears probably devoted 3 to 4 hours a day to activities they needed to sustain themselves. The rest of the time, they laid back and had a good time.

When's the last time you did the same? If you're like most men, you're almost drowning in stress. Consider what stress does to your body. Let's say you had a miserable day at the office. This kind of short-term stress has been found to reduce bloodflow to the penis and testicles and send testosterone into freefall. Then there's long-term, or chronic, stress. It has the same unpleasant effects as short-term stress, multiplied by a lot. Men who live a pressure-cooker existence tend to have low libido and fertility. They're more likely to accumulate blood-blocking deposits on tiny blood vessels in the penis. They're also more likely to slide into depression.

It's almost impossible to have good sex when you're stressed. Sex, after all, requires time, energy, and cooperation between (at least) two people. A man who's stressed will find it difficult to achieve even one of these elements, let alone all of them.

We'll talk in detail about techniques for managing stress in just a bit. For now, it's enough to say that you have to recognize what's happening to you. Do you have trouble concentrating? Get enraged at minor inconveniences, like getting cut off in traffic by the moron in the BMW? Have trouble sleeping? Feel an emptiness in the pit of your stomach, as though you're getting gnawed by rodents? Stress affects us all to some degree, and it's essential to apply the brakes before it takes over your life.

Forget any advice that starts with something like, "Eliminate the stress in your life." Can't do it. Stress is everywhere. It's part of our world, and the only way to eliminate it is to live in a cave some-where—and even then you'd probably get stressed about spiders. You might not be able to hide from stress, but you can always manage it.

Exercise, obviously, is a great stress reducer. Studies have shown that men who get as little as 30 minutes of regular moderate exer-cise have dramatic declines in stress levels and a corresponding in-crease in endorphins, the brain chemicals that produce feelings of well-being. In fact, researchers at Duke University have shown that exercising for 30 minutes a day three or four times a week can be as effective as prescription antidepressants at relieving symptoms of anxiety and depression. Even if you do nothing more vigorous than taking your dog for a daily walk, you'll have a drop in blood pres-sure, more flexible muscles, and an increase in bloodflow to tissues throughout your body, including the penis, where it's needed for erections.

DEPRESSION

It's among the most stealthy, and potentially devastating, conditions that men face. Don't believe the stereotypes. Most men with de-pression don't spend their days holed up in dark rooms contem-plating "the big jump." They don't quit their jobs or quit talking to family and friends. On the surface, men with depression often ap-pear fine—but inside they feel lost and hopeless and drained of life.

The scary thing about depression is how gradually it can take over your life. You probably won't recognize what's happening at first. As the months go by, you might find yourself sleeping a little more, avoiding people you used to spend time with, or slipping a little bit at work. Given enough time, depression will start hammering away at more and more of your life until you can hardly remember feeling energized and excited by—well, just about anything.

Sex is often the first casualty. Men who are depressed typically have little interest in sex or even masturbation. You aren't going to feel very sexy when your mood is in the basement, and you might not have the energy to think about dating or starting a relationship. Even if you do find yourself (or already are) with a partner, you'll probably have trouble getting erections—a classic sign of depression. At the same time, of course, trouble in the bedroom is almost certain to make your mood and self-esteem worse.

Depression is a disease. As soon as you recognize the symptoms—trouble sleeping, a loss of interest in things that used to please you, changes in your eating or sleeping habits, excessive anger, and so on—you have to get help. Start with a therapist. Or see your regular doctor. Depression is hardly an arcane, hard-to-diagnose condition. Doctors see a lot of men with depression, and they can usually spot the signs right away.

The usual treatment these days, along with counseling, is antidepressants. Take advantage of them. These drugs aren't for everyone, but they've turned things around for millions of men. Yes, some drugs cause sexual side effects, mainly erection problems or loss of libido. Don't let this keep you from getting treatment. For one thing, while anywhere from 20 to 37 percent of men who take these drugs will have sexual side effects, many others don't. With some of the newer drugs, such as Lexapro (escitalopram), this number drops to the low single digits. The consequences of untreated depression are far more severe than anything you're likely to experience from treatment.

Incidentally, some men find that the sexual side effects are reduced when they take the antidepressant early in the day. In addition, men who take antidepressants often have dramatic improvement in their sex lives when they add Viagra or one of the newer erection drugs to the mix. University of New Mexico researchers gave Viagra or a placebo to 76 men on antidepressants who complained of sexual problems such as low sex drive and erection difficulties. Those who took Viagra for 6 weeks reported significantly improved libidos, erections, ejaculation, and overall sexual satisfaction.

While you're getting help—or sooner if you recognize the signs—find the strength in yourself to be physically active. Antidepressants can take weeks or months to work, but exercise kicks in immediately. The changes in brain chemistry that accompany even a half-hearted workout will give you a nearly instant mood lift. It won't eliminate depression, but it can pull you up a few notches and make it easier to pursue other options, such as therapy, that will get you on your feet again. Definitely consider activities that involve other people, such as team sports or a cardiovascular conditioning class, like Spinning or Tae Bo. Depression is invariably accompanied by loneliness and a sense of isolation. Spending time with others can provide the little spark that you need to keep going.

FOCUS ON BETTER SEX

Sex has relatively little to do with the few square inches of anatomy below your belt. Whether you're a once-a-week kind of guy or a twice-every-day dynamo, your libido is inextricably linked to your mental and emotional health. If you're stressed all the time, you might as well say goodbye to sex. The same with persistent insomnia, depression, or anything else that puts you off your game.

These are huge issues, of course, and every man has to choose his own weapons to fight back. In nearly all cases, though, one of the most powerful tools is meditation. If you're like most of us, you've probably given little thought to it. Not many men do, now that the '60s are 40 years gone. The average American man takes a serious look at meditation only when a particularly luscious lover practically insists on it.

Forget all the spiritual components of meditation. Let's consider it from an American's point of view: It offers huge returns with minimal investments. Better yet, you can do it without much effort. Simply sitting down and breathing easily once a day for 10 to 30 minutes will increase energy and lung capacity, lower blood pressure, tune up your nervous system, and yes, put you in the mental place where sex is once again a pleasure.

Those are just the physical benefits. Meditation helps you think clearly and keep your cool. It balances the physical, emotional, and mental parts of your personality. It puts you in harmony—a New Age–y way of saying that it makes you strong and focused. Strong men feel sexy and are *very* sexy to women.

With meditation, in other words, your life gets better. So yeah, it deserves a closer look. There are probably dozens of styles of mediation. Forget about chanting, om-ing, or sitting in uncomfortable positions on the floor. That's all eye candy. Meditation, at its core, doesn't require anything more complicated than a willingness to relax, listen to your body, and let your mind drift.

THE POWER OF BREATHING

Let's take a closer look at what happens physically during meditation. It's not all that different from the benefits you get from working out, minus the sweat.

Picture a guy in a chair doing nothing. Maybe he even has his eyes closed. Or he might be staring dreamily into space. First impression: "What a loser."

Take a closer look. He's doing more than you might think. Notice his chest rising and falling in perfect rhythm. He looks like he's sleeping, but wait—he isn't drooling, and his head isn't falling on his chest. In fact, he looks calm, at peace with himself, even powerful in a self-possessed kind of way.

Now, imagine what's happening inside his body. With every breath, the muscles between the ribs contract. The diaphragm, that dome-shaped muscle sitting on top of the stomach, moves down and opens up more space for the lungs. The heart is pumping calmly, pushing a stream of oxygen-poor blood into the lungs for refreshment. Fatigue-causing carbon dioxide gets pushed out, while life-supporting oxygen floods through the body's cells and stimulates the release of calming endorphins.

In short, all of that "doing nothing" is like a jolt of pure sexual juice. The muscles are loading up with oxygen and glycogen, the sugar they need for fuel. The endocrine system is functioning at optimal levels, producing and secreting sex and other hormones at the precise times they're needed. The brain is churning out alpha waves—low-energy spikes of electrical activity that indicate serenity. Your whole body, when you meditate, enters a state that doctors call wakeful relaxation. In less clinical terms, you're almost as high as a kite.

The point of all this is to show that breathing isn't simply what you do to stay alive. It's an essential component of mental as well as physical health. Most of us, because we live lives of almost chronic stress, don't breathe very naturally or efficiently. If anything, we pant like tired dogs on a hot day, taking rapid, shallow breaths that keep us functional, but not much more. Bad breathing means nervousness and tension. It means tight muscles and high blood pressure. Most of all, it means we have almost a screaming need for more oxygen—not just occasionally, but all the time.

Wonder why your sex life isn't what it could be? Better

breathing—and with it, an increase in confidence and well-being—can be part of the answer.

That's why you need to meditate. It's the simplest thing in the world, so don't make it harder than it has to be. Don't worry about emptying your mind or finding your third eye or whatever. Just pay attention to your breathing. Here's how to do it.

RELAX–REALLY RELAX. Most of us tighten up when we're trying to do anything, even if that means doing nothing. You've got to fight that impulse. Sit in a comfortable chair. Put both feet flat on the floor. Relax your shoulders, your hands and arms. Close your eyes and breathe as naturally as you know how: deeply and regularly, in and out.

At this point, you're probably so intent on breathing *naturally* that all your muscles are fighting back. You've probably managed to tighten your biceps, squeeze your shoulders up, and clench your jaw. You need to relax here. Start again.

TRACK YOUR BREATHING. With each inhalation, notice how the air feels going in. Is it reaching only as far as your chest, or do you get the sense that it's pouring into the bottommost levels of your lungs? It's a subtle difference, but you can feel it when it's right.

▼

Is lovemaking good for your skin? It is if you suffer from dermatitis, a condition characterized by outbreaks of rashes and blemishes. Getting hot and sweaty during sex flushes skin pores and helps prevent inflammation.

▲

GO DEEP. Fill your lungs completely with each breath. This means breathing slowly, with your muscles as relaxed as they can get. Then exhale, slowly and completely. Are you relaxed and naturally allowing your body to do what it's designed to do? Or are you tensing your muscles because you're determined to do it right? Remember, this is all about letting go and not forcing anything. You'll know you're doing it right when you stop thinking about each breath, when you don't feel that you *need* extra oxygen.

TAKE THE 30-SECOND BREATH TEST. If you want to see if you're really breathing right, lie down the next time to try this. Put a lightweight object such as a box of tissues on top of your abdomen. If it gently rises and falls as you breathe, you'll know you're pulling oxygen as deeply as it's meant to go. If the object doesn't move at all, on the other hand, you're still breathing too shallowly.

KEEP IT SIMPLE. Meditating with deep breathing is so simple that it's hard to believe anything is happening—and you'll probably be tempted to do something *extra*. This usually means breathing faster than you need to. Resist the impulse. Fast breathing totally disrupts the balance of carbon dioxide and oxygen. It will make you more stressed, not less. Remember, less is more: Let your breathing happen naturally. Be aware of it and let it happen. Don't interfere with it.

CALL IT GOOD AFTER ABOUT 10 MINUTES. Congratulations. You've just meditated. Really, that's all there is to it. If you give yourself time to do this exercise a couple of times a day, paying attention to your breathing but not really forcing anything, you'll naturally feel more energized. Your levels of stress hormones will drop, not only during the meditation but also for hours afterward. You'll feel more confident because you'll have better control of your body. And that control naturally translates into better health, better living, better sex. In half an hour or less a day.

PICTURE PLEASURE

When you first start to meditate, or on days when your brain feels like it's crammed with screaming demons, you'll find that you're too distracted to just sit and let go. This happens to everyone. With a little practice, you'll learn to shut down the mind noise and slip into relaxed, quiet breathing as easily as sliding into a hot tub.

But when life is really crazy, you might want to add another component to your meditation sessions—a component that's even easier than breathing because it requires nothing more than filling your mind with mood-changing scenes.

CREATE A MENTAL PICTURE. Close your eyes and imagine that you're standing in a pristine forest clearing. It's green, quiet, private. Maybe you're sitting on a rock, your back warmed by the sun. You can feel a light breeze brushing your skin, and you can hear the rustle of leaves. You haven't moved from your chair, but your mind is somewhere else altogether. It's in a place where you feel totally and blissfully relaxed. (Don't fight it; just do it.)

GIVE YOUR EMOTIONS SHAPE. As you drift deeper and deeper into the scene, you'll notice other thoughts creeping in—the stresses of the day, for example, or conflicts you've had at home or work. Don't dwell on the thoughts themselves. Instead, imagine that each thought, and the stress that it represents, is an animal that's crept into your mental dreamscape. For example, imagine that the blinking light on your telephone (maybe a message from your landlord?) is a dog in the forest, sniffing the air. Anxiety about loose ends at work? Turn it into a garter snake winding through the grass. An argument with your wife? It becomes a raccoon.

Now, wait a bit to see what else approaches. When no more thought-animals appear, mentally stand up and walk around the clearing. Approach the animals. Acknowledge their presence, but don't dwell on what they represent. Touch them one by one—and imagine that with your touch, they amble out of the clearing.

COME BACK TO SOLITUDE. You're alone again after all the animals, all your cares, have left the scene. Return to the rock, the sunshine, the rustle of leaves. Breathe deeply and quietly for 10 minutes, focusing on your breath the way you did before. Then stand up, stretch, and return to the present.

Psychologists call this process visualization. It's a way of taking your mind out of the stressful present. More important, it allows you to acknowledge all the things that are bothering you without giving them the power to disrupt your mental peace.

Researchers have been studying visualization for decades. Research at top universities has shown that visualization dramatically decreases stress, improves your ability to focus, and even strengthens the immune system. Two such studies found that stressed-out medical students who used visualization techniques at exam times had fewer viral infections. Another study found that patients who had recurrent bouts of genital herpes cut their outbreaks in half and boosted their natural killer cell activity when they did visualization. It has even been used to relieve impotence in some men. You can also use visualization to have better sex. That's not as surprising as it might sound. After all, we all know that hot thoughts prime us for sex long before the event. When you spend an evening with someone you like, with lots of laughing, talking, flirting, and touching, your mind and body are preparing for sex, whether you're conscious of it or not.

If you still don't buy into conjuring up little animal friends, consider the science behind visualization: Visual and tactile images stimulate the part of the brain responsible for language, thinking, and problem solving. When researchers used sophisticated brain-scanning tools to monitor the brain while people were visualizing something, they found that the same part of the brain was activated whether the person was merely imagining something or actually experiencing it.

You can use the process to minimize romance-busting distractions and enhance your erotic mental space.

▶ Breathe deeply for 5 minutes or so. When you're thoroughly relaxed, close your eyes and imagine that you and your partner are standing a few feet apart. You're both enclosed in a bubble of golden light.

▶ Picture a blue light, about the size of a soccer ball, hovering in front of your partner. The ball is a magnet, one that attracts anything bad: old arguments, tension between you, whatever.

▶ Let the ball hang in the air as long as necessary to fill itself up with all of life's nastiness. When there's nothing left, imagine the ball hurtling out into space and exploding into smithereens.

▶ Now imagine that anyone who could potentially come between the two of you—say, the guy you hate who flirts with her at work—has come into your private little bubble. Tell him to get lost. Picture him fading out of the bubble.

▶ Now you're alone, the two of you. Imagine that there's a gold sphere hanging in the air. Give it a characteristic that you'd both like to share, such as love, comfort, or creative sexual energy. Watch as the gold melts and coats the walls of your bubble, surrounding you with all you want to experience.

Hold the thought for a few minutes, take a few deep breaths, then open your eyes. All of those visual thoughts are now implanted in your brain—and we all know the power of suggestion. You'll feel sexier and more erotically charged. Both your mind and body are now primed because you've essentially created a new reality.

Sound crazy? Maybe it does, but visualization has worked for thousands of test subjects—in fact, it's been estimated that it could offer help for some 90 percent of the problems that send people to their doctors. And it will work for you.

REKINDLE THE FLAMES
Our cultural landscape is littered with jokes about wives who avoid sex with their husbands. The line, "Not tonight, dear, I've got a

headache," doesn't even need a reference to sex for us to know exactly what's being said.

There are certainly plenty of wives who don't want to have sex with their husbands. What you might not know is that it's often the man who isn't putting out. In fact, psychologists who specialize in couples' therapy say that low libido, sometimes called inhibited desire syndrome, is among the chief complaints that married men put on the table.

Each couple is different, just as each man and woman is different. There's rarely a single reason to explain the damping of the fire. Certainly, fatigue and stress are among the main reasons that many married men have little or no sex. American life places so many pressures on couples that they depend more on antidepressants than on each other. A man who comes home exhausted from work will be hard-pressed to find the energy to be intimate.

The problem often lies less with the man than with the dynamics of the marriage itself. Couples who aren't happy with each other, who spend an inordinate number of their waking hours harboring resentments about one thing or another, are unlikely to spend time heating up the sheets. Even in a marriage that's otherwise happy, men and women can get so used to each other that they no longer feel those delicious thrills. They get bored, in other words.

When the spark of love is first kindled, people can't get enough of each other. They adore everything, and faults are perceived as small or even endearing. And so, off to the chapel they go, the perfect couple, perfectly united, till death do they part.

Then the years go by, and many a husband or wife decides they've had quite enough, thank you. Instead of a perfect couple, perfectly united, they find themselves sadly limping along.

Many marriages are on the whole quite happy even when sex is lacking. But most men and women would welcome more sexual intimacy. The challenge is to find ways to fan the embers so that you

MALE MENOPAUSE: FACT OR MYTH?

A man's production of testosterone and other sex hormones declines with age—and after your mid-40s, the drop can be dramatic. That's precisely when a man's sex drive and ability to have erections also wane. This has led some researchers to speculate that men experience *andropause,* the male equivalent of menopause.

The possibility that men experience a winding down of their reproductive potential is sharply debated among experts. Believers point out that testosterone, which is critical for male sexual function, starts dropping precipitously at about age 45, the age when many men start reporting impotence and low libido, along with such things as depression, mood swings, and even hot flashes. They also note that there's an age-related increase in a blood protein that latches onto sex hormones and essentially takes them out of service. The amount of *available* testosterone in a man's blood may drop by as much as 50 percent between the ages of 25 and 75.

Skeptics—and most medical doctors fall into this camp—contend that there's no evidence that normal declines in testosterone have any effect on libido. Further, so-called age-related testosterone drops may in fact be caused by other things, such as testicular inflammation, obesity, diabetes, or too much alcohol. A man who starts having erection problems could very well have underlying medical problems that have nothing to do with testosterone. Diet may even play a role. A study at the University of Massachusetts Medical School involving 1,522 men ages 40 to 70 found that protein-deficient diets led to decreased testosterone activity, which in turn caused declines in sexual performance.

Even if you don't have any specific health problems, you might notice a decline in sexual performance if you're generally out of shape—smoking too much, drinking too much, and so on. Whether or not there turns out to be such a thing as andropause, nearly every man will benefit, in and out of the bedroom, just by getting back in shape. Basic lifestyle changes—eating a healthful diet, exercising regularly, giving up the smokes, and drinking in moderation—will probably do more for your sex life than taking a boatload of hormones.

can experience the delicious heat once again—assuming you even want to.

That's a key point. If you no longer feel sexual desire for your partner, you have some real thinking to do. At the very least, you have to decide if the "problem"—assuming it is a problem for the two of you—is one that you're willing to take the time and effort to work out.

START WITH A CHECKUP. There are dozens of physical problems that can sap libido and the ability to have erections. Diabetes and thyroid disease, for example, are among the most common diseases doctors treat, and both can take a heavy toll on desire. So can the use of prescription drugs, especially sedatives and antidepressants.

BE MORE THAN A SOCCER DAD. It's normal for couples to get so preoccupied with the stresses of daily life—work, raising children, struggling to pay the bills—that they simply don't have any energy left for each other. Relationships can chug along for decades without any real intimacy, but is that what you really want? Even if sex isn't a top priority for you—and for many men as well as women, it doesn't even make the top 10—you'd probably enjoy more closeness and intimacy.

It simply isn't possible to vacuum all of the stress out of your life. That said, there are always ways to open up the time and space to relax and enjoy each other again. This might mean insisting that your kids give up at least one of their extracurricular activities, such as soccer or karate. Or designate one night a week a TV-free night. You might even decide to turn down a promotion that will only add more hours to an already stressful week. Good sex takes time, and the time spent in bed is the least of it. It's the time you spend together day to day that makes the biggest difference.

TAKE AN EMOTIONAL READING. Are you angry, hurt, resentful? Do you feel taken for granted, ignored? If so, speak up. Allowing such feelings to fester is not a solution. You have to stand up for yourself, to make sure your partner understands what you need. Counseling—with a therapist who specializes in marriage issues or simply with a wise friend—is among the most important steps you can take.

Of course, you may look into yourself and decide that your feelings, sexual and otherwise, are really and truly gone—and decide that it's time to abandon this foundering, sexless ship. But before you make that decision and find yourself awash in lawyers and the truly devastating fact of divorce, try to remember all of the things that drew you to your partner in the first place. She was the light of your life—remember? The first one you thought of every morning when you woke up, and the one who was in your mind as you drifted off to sleep each night. Remember that woman? She might still be there for you. It's worth making every effort to rediscover her for yourself.

CHAPTER **13**

PERFORMANCE PROBLEMS

**IF YOU HAVEN'T CHEWED YOUR NAILS BECAUSE OF
SEXUAL PROBLEMS OF ONE KIND OR ANOTHER, YOU'RE
CERTAINLY NOT MALE, AND POSSIBLY NOT EVEN HUMAN.**
We *all* worry about performance on occasion, sometimes with good
reason. Maybe you didn't get hard with a new partner, despite all
the sexy foreplay. Maybe you tend to come quicker than you want.
Or maybe you just worry in general, because, let's face it, sex carries a lot of freight. None of us wants to be judged harshly in that
emotion-packed arena.

Low sex drive, performance anxiety, premature ejaculation, impotence. For millions of men, these aren't just theoretical possi-
bilities, but a very real part of lovemaking. Like it or not, your
body isn't a machine. Even if you're generally happy with your
sexual performance, there will be times when the gears stop
turning—because you're nervous, trying too hard to please, or
maybe just had too much to drink. Your mind is willing, your

partner is willing, but your body says, "Nope." Embarrassing? You bet.

The embarrassment, and the accompanying crash in self-esteem and confidence, is magnified when sexual difficulties are starting to define your relationships. Millions of men—tens of millions, actually—have persistent problems with erections, low libido, or too-quick ejaculation. The cliché "misery loves company" isn't really true. But you can take some comfort in the fact that the things you're dealing with are understood very well by doctors and therapists—and yes, by women, too. If you're honest and open about what's happening, you're a lot more likely to get patient sympathy than rejection. Besides, the sexual problems we're talking about are precisely the ones that are easiest to change.

Most sexual problems, whether physical or psychological—they're usually a complicated mix of the two—run in packs. A man whose sex drive has dropped, for example, might experience erection problems as well. Obviously, there are probably hundreds of reasons for sexual disappointment and just as much variation in their manifestations and severity.

Keep this point in mind: Sexual letdowns are *normal*. Once you reach your 40s, erections will probably take their sweet time arriving, and they might flag almost as soon as you've started. Your sex drive is undoubtedly lower than it used to be, and your orgasms aren't as intense as you remember. *"During my late 30s (I'm now 41), I noticed a decrease in my libido,"* one man told us. *"I think stress and depression contributed to that."*

He's probably right. Lifestyle pressures play an enormous role in sexual satisfaction. If you're stressed in your life, that stress is going to show up in bed. Even if you're having good sex most of the time, there will certainly be nights when you'll fail because you're too balled up to relax. Depression, anxiety about sex, or just garden-variety stress can combine with normal (or not so normal) physical issues and really shut you down.

Forget embarrassment. Forget silent suffering. Sexual insecurity plagues way too many men—men who could turn things around if they'd only find the strength in themselves to face up to the issues, step up to the plate, and get the help they need.

WHEN LIBIDO IS LACKING

You've probably heard the expression, "Women need a reason to have sex; men only need a place." The implicit message is that men *always* want sex, are *always* hard, are *always* willing. With this kind of cultural (and misleading) hype filling our heads, it's hardly surprising that our sexual expectations are always butting heads with sexual reality.

It's almost meaningless to talk about normal sex drive, because there's no such thing. Maybe you want to have sex two or even three times a day, every day. Good for you. Or maybe you want it once a week or once a month or once a *year*. Again, good for you—if you and your partner are happy. Granted, a man who happily waits a year between trysts would raise eyebrows in just about any company, but the point is the same. Libido isn't some absolute that can be measured with scales and plotted on an Ideal Frequency Chart. All scientists can do is pass out survey forms, tally up the answers, and determine that the average man has sex with X amount of frequency. That doesn't mean that X is the gold standard or that guys who fall below or above the average are in any way abnormal.

Since there isn't really such a thing as a normal libido, how do you know if yours is lower than it should be (or you want it to be)? Specialists in male sexuality are interested mainly in any *changes* you've experienced—and whether or not you're satisfied with the level of your sexual interest. A man who used to want sex three times a week and suddenly wants it a lot less probably has some issues to deal with. The same with a man who's having conflicts with his partner because the amount of sex he wants doesn't jibe with her desires.

All sorts of things can take the steam out of libido. Here are some of the main ones.

▶ **Age**. Most men desire less sex as they get older. This might be related to natural declines in testosterone. It can also be a function of experience: A man's who's been having sex for decades is less likely to be over-the-top sex crazy than a man who's had fewer opportunities to indulge.

▶ **Illness**. It's a very common cause of low libido. If you don't feel well physically, you're not going to be in the mood for sex. Related to this is the use of prescription drugs. Low libido is a common side effect of blood pressure drugs, antidepressants, and many others.

▶ **Boredom**. If you've been in the same relationship for a long time, it's natural to get a little blasé about sex. You might take each other for granted or find each other so predictable that the sizzle is gone.

▶ **Insecurity and uncertainty**. Men who have had rough sexual experiences—for example, criticism about their bodies from past partners—may simply give up because they find sex too threatening.

▶ **Stress**. This is the big one. If you're weighed down by the pressures of the world—work issues, money issues, kid issues—your sexual energy is going to take a hit. The greater the stress, the lower your libido is likely to be.

Low libido isn't necessarily a huge issue in a man's life, especially if he's with a partner whose sexual expectations match his own. What often happens, though, is that libido gradually declines over months or years. The tapering occurs so slowly that you're hardly aware of it—until one day your lover looks at you and says something like, "We hardly ever make love anymore. Don't you desire me?"

Pay attention to those words. What she's telling you is that the two of you are out of sync—and the next step could be a divorce lawyer if you don't take a hard look at what's happening.

There aren't any quick-and-easy solutions because the causes of low libido vary so much. But if your sex drive is lower than you'd like, there are a few things you'll probably want to try.

CHECK THE FLUIDS. If your libido is lower than it used to be—maybe you only want sex every few weeks and used to crave it almost every day—you have to make sure that there isn't an underlying medical problem behind it. Some men, for example, do have low levels of testosterone. Taking a synthetic hormone could jump-start desire in dramatic ways. *"Testosterone replacement—fantastic! Fantastic!"* a 58-year-old retired educator told us. *"I noticed an increase in libido within days. I also had more energy and a better sense of well-being."*

SNEAK AWAY FROM WORK. Okay, you can let your boss know ahead of time, but still get away. Take a real day off, and do it as often as you can. Stress is probably the number one killer of sex drive, and as you get older, your levels of responsibilities and obligations will only get heavier. You have to cut yourself the slack to *live,* not just stagger from one duty to the next.

Stress takes a lot of different forms, but the techniques for beating it—exercise, meditation, yoga, volunteer work, whatever works for you—are pretty much the same. Once you give yourself a little mental and physical R&R, you'll find that your energy for all things, including sex, rises fast.

PUMP UP YOUR CHEMISTRY. Okay, you already know that exercise makes you look better and feel better. And it can have

THE SEXUAL FOUNTAIN OF YOUTH

A 1999 survey of 3,500 people found that those who had sex at least three times a week tended to look up to 10 years younger than those who had sex less often. Other surveys report that men and women who look younger than their chronological ages had sex 50 percent more often than those who looked their age.

Researchers speculate that frequent sex increases levels of hormones that reduce fatty tissue and increase lean muscle, giving a more youthful appearance.

significant effects on your libido. Men who exercise feel better about their bodies. That's as close to a natural aphrodisiac as you can get. Exercise also increases levels of endorphins, brain chemicals that make you feel good. At the same time, it lowers levels of stress hormones and improves your ability to focus and relax.

FIND YOUR EROTIC TRIGGERS. Sex is such emotionally charged terrain that many of us play it safe. We learn certain styles of foreplay or sexual positions when we're young and keep doing the same things year after year. There's nothing wrong with staying in your comfort zone—when it's working. But if you find that your erotic energy isn't as charged as you like, you might need the stimulation that comes from doing something different. Are you usually quiet during sex? Launch into some sexy talk—as dirty as you like—and encourage your partner to do the same. Play with massage oils or sex toys. Fill your head with fantasies and excite your partner with the details.

These examples might not really float your boat, of course. Experiment until you find what does. Your libido might be perfectly normal, but maybe you've never taken the time to identify the sexual triggers that really work for you.

TALK WITH YOUR PARTNER. Do it. Talk about issues that scare you, issues that make you angry, resentments you've probably buried as deep as they'll go. Couples who stop having sex often have some serious issues to discuss or at least some petty annoyances that no one's talking about. Couples' therapy is an obvious place to start. At the very least, set aside an hour just to clear the air. You don't need a clear agenda, just the desire to talk about whatever comes to mind.

If you do it right, without being defensive or accusatory, you may find out some surprising things about each other, including sexual desires and preferences that you haven't talked about before—and that can supercharge a relationship that has gotten a little tired.

FEAR ON CENTER STAGE

"Will I get hard in time?" "Hope she isn't put off by this extra weight." "What if I come too fast?" "I'm not staying hard—damn, it's getting limp." "I'm not sure she likes what I'm doing."

Welcome to the world of mind-messing mental monologues that almost guarantee you won't get it up—or even if you do, will make it hard to enjoy yourself fully. You can't have good sex, or any sex in some cases, when you're fixated on your own performance.

Every man and woman gets anxious with a new partner. If you've had sexual difficulties in the past, terrified might be closer to the mark. When the two of you get undressed and climb into bed, do all of your anxieties rustle around in your brain like squirrels in a sack?

Your body responds to anxiety. It interprets it as a perceived threat, then does what evolution programmed it to do: It releases chemicals called catecholamines, which trigger the fight-or-flight response. What this means, among other things, is that your body protects vital organs with more blood, while depriving less important areas (you can guess which) of the blood they need. To put it simply, your heart and lungs take precedence over a dozing penis. Never mind that blood is precisely what you want down there at this anxious juncture; your body has other plans for the stuff.

Performance anxiety isn't the same as full-fledged impotence. A man whose machinery is in perfect working order can still succumb. If you're lucky, it won't be anything worse than a now-and-then embarrassment. The danger is that previous failures to get an erection will fill your mind with so much stress that future failures are all but certain. The prophecy becomes self-fulfilling. And in the worst case, you might helplessly watch as your relationship deteriorates because your partner is convinced that what's happening with your penis is a sign of what's happening in your mind—that you don't love her or find her attractive.

More than a few men cope with performance anxiety simply by avoiding sex. Obviously, that's not much of a coping mechanism. If anything, it makes things worse because your partner will naturally assume you're rejecting her. Then the demons of insecurity will start prodding *her*. She might start avoiding sex herself. Even if she's not angry or resentful, she might say no just to spare you embarrassment.

Performance anxiety can and does escalate, so you want to take positive action the first time it occurs. Here's what experts advise.

OWN UP TO IT. You're a man, right? That means that anything short of a spear in the chest will be met with artful denial. Get over it. If you're not getting hard because you're nervous, say so. Tell her what you'd like her to do—even if that means doing nothing at the moment. Pretending that everything's fine won't fool her anyway, and it will reinforce in your own mind the idea that you have something to be ashamed of. Any woman who's spent time in the real world knows about performance anxiety. She'll be sympathetic, not shocked. *"Communication is everything,"* a 40-year-old woman told us. *"Talk about it, work it out together."*

TAKE YOUR MIND OFF YOUR PENIS. Take your hands off it, too, and ask her to do the same. Once the anxiety of getting an erection sets in, trying to force things will only make you more anxious, so forget about it for awhile. Massage her, touch her, play with her. Let her play with you (but not there). Drink a glass of wine and talk for awhile. Once you're relaxed and thinking about other things, there's a good chance that you'll get back in form.

FORGET INTERCOURSE. If performance anxiety keeps raising its ugly head, you might want to give up on intercourse for a little while, long enough to shift your focus, and hers, away from your penis. Tell her what's happening. Be totally straight and suggest that the two of you have different kinds of sex for awhile. Once your penis isn't the centerpiece of lovemaking, you won't have to worry that it won't get hard. It might, and it might not. It won't matter, because the two of you will be doing other things that are equally entertaining. In the meantime, you'll have less to worry about. When you find you're consistently getting an erection during sex and foreplay, then by all means, have at it.

LAUGH ABOUT IT. Okay, it isn't very funny at the moment. But put things in perspective: Men have been getting nervous about sex since long before you were born, and they'll be getting nervous long after you're gone. You know it; your partner knows it. It's just an *erection,* for God's sake! Let it take care of itself. It will come back once the worry's on a back burner.

NOT HARD ENOUGH

For some men, impotence comes and goes. For others, it's a lifelong curse. Either way, it's a lot like the IRS—sooner or later, it's bound to catch up with you.

Doctors estimate that about 15 percent of American men suffer from this supremely frustrating problem, also known as erectile dysfunction. It generally starts happening when a man reaches his 40s. In that age group, about 4 in 10 men experience it to some degree. By the time men hit their 70s, the percentage jumps to 70 percent.

Doctors define erectile dysfunction as the repeated inability to get or keep an erection firm enough for intercourse. It can happen whether or not you're aroused. The occasional bout of impotence isn't worth discussing with your doctor, but if it's happening often or all the time, you definitely want to talk to someone.

All sorts of things can cause erection problems. Here are the main ones.

▶ Underlying health problems. About 70 percent of all cases have a physical origin, ranging from diabetes or vascular disease to hypertension.

▶ Prescription or over-the-counter drugs. Antidepressants, sedatives, blood pressure drugs, and antihistamines are all common culprits. There are many others besides.

▶ Depression or anxiety. These and other mental or emotional problems play a key role in anywhere from 10 to 30 percent of cases and are probably involved to some extent in a much greater percentage.

Since the ability to have sex cuts so close to the core of a man's sense of self, persistent problems can be devastating. Most men, unfortunately, tend to look the other way. They know what's happening, they see the effects impotence has on their partners as well as themselves, but they can't bring themselves to face it squarely. That's unfortunate because current treatments—often a combination of counseling and drugs, and in some cases, surgery—are extremely effective. In addition, recent studies suggest that the earlier a man begins dealing with erection problems, the better his odds of making a complete recovery. Here are some of your options.

WALK FOR BETTER SEX. No kidding. Even though vigorous exercise such as lifting weights or swimming can help restore libido as well as erections, all you really have to do is walk a couple of miles a day. Doctors at the New England Research Institute found that men who burned an extra 200 calories a day—the equivalent of walking 2 miles—were far less likely to experience impotence than those who were sedentary. The prestigious *British Medical Journal* recently reported that men over the age of 50 who stay physically active are 30 percent less likely to experience impotence than those who are inactive.

Men who are physically active also report better erections and seem to have the sexual abilities of men 2 to 5 years younger.

GET YOUR LIFE UNDER CONTROL. You're probably tired of hearing it, but giving up smoking, staying lean, and drinking moderately can vastly improve your chances of staying sexually healthy. Even if you're already having problems, straightening out your life will improve the circulation that you need for good erections.

ASK ABOUT VIAGRA. Men with impaired bloodflow due to accumulations of fatty crud on arteries in the penis—which, after about the age of 40 or 50, applies to nearly all men to some degree—can get dramatic improvement by taking Viagra, Levitra, or Cialis, drugs that cause blood vessels to relax and engorge with blood.

About 80 percent of men who take these drugs report a significant improvement in their ability to get erections. As a bonus, the erections are usually harder than they were before.

Viagra and related drugs do have side effects—mainly headaches, facial flushing, or congestion—but they're safe for the vast majority of men. The exception is if you have heart problems or are taking nitrate drugs, in which case Viagra is probably too dangerous to use.

INJECT FOR BETTER SEX. If oral drugs don't work for you, your doctor might advise using an injectable drug, such as papaverine, phentolamine, or alprostadil (marketed as Caverject). Injected into the penis prior to sex, these drugs widen blood vessels and almost instantly promote erections. They aren't used very often because they frequently cause side effects, including scarring of the penis. They can also cause a *painfully* persistent erection, a condition called priapism.

RUB YOURSELF RIGHT. The drug nitroglycerine, used in cream form, will sometimes enhance an erection when rubbed on the penis prior to sex.

GET A TESTOSTERONE BOOST. If you have low levels of natural testosterone, your doctor might advise you to use a testosterone-replacement patch. Most men with erection problems have normal levels of testosterone, so this treatment isn't used very often. But if you're truly deficient in testosterone, hormone therapy might be part of the answer.

PUSH THE PELLET. A drug delivery system marketed as Muse is used to insert a tiny pellet of a drug called alprostadil into the urethra, the opening in the penis. You should start getting an erection in about 10 minutes. The drug is very effective, but side effects, including aching in the penis or testicles or irritation in the urethra, are common.

SUCK IT UP. You can buy vacuum pumps from medical supply stores and Internet sources. You insert your penis into a plastic tube prior to sex, then use a hand pump to create a vacuum that pulls blood into the penis and causes an erection. The blood is kept in place by placing a flexible ring around the base of the penis.

Vacuum pumps aren't exactly romantic, and they do interrupt the normal sexual flow, but they work. If you go this route, remember to remove the rubber ring from your penis within about 30 minutes to restore normal circulation.

CONSIDER THE SURGICAL ROUTE. This isn't an option doctors take lightly, and neither should you. Once you have surgery for erection problems, there's no going back; you'll never get natural erections again. But for men with vascular or nerve disease, who are unable to get erections naturally, the surgery can be little less than a miracle.

Doctors use a number of different techniques. Probably the most common is to implant inflatable rods into the penis. When you're ready for sex, you squeeze a bulb inside the scrotum to pump up the rods. Your penis gets hard, you have sex, and then you make an adjustment that allows the rods to deflate.

Anything with moveable parts has the potential to break down, of course. Some men decide to trade high-tech convenience for something a little more reliable, such as semi-rigid rods. In essence, they give you a sort of permanent erection—hard enough for sex, but not so rigid that it's embarrassingly visible through your khakis at work.

QUICK ON THE TRIGGER

Premature ejaculation, like beauty, is entirely in the eyes of the beholder. If you come within 30 seconds of starting intercourse, and you and your partner are satisfied, well, it was obviously long enough. If you last so long that you can listen to most of a Norah Jones CD, but you and your partner still want more, that's premature—at least for you.

Satisfaction is at the heart of any definition of premature ejaculation. As a general rule, if you come too fast to satisfy yourself or your partner, you'll want to do something about it.

"Premature ejaculation is the bane of my existence," said a 41-year-old information technology project manager who responded to our survey. *"I always orgasm very quickly, anywhere from 30 seconds to 2 minutes after entering my wife. It makes me very frustrated because I love the feeling of my penis inside her vagina during intercourse."*

MIND OVER ORGASM

Men have come up with all sorts of tactics for delaying the explosion into orgasm: thinking about baseball, visualizing scenes from a Stephen King movie, or in extreme cases, imagining a Barry Manilow song. Can you really stop yourself from coming with mental distraction alone?

Not likely. When your body is seconds away from an orgasmic crescendo, nothing that floats through your mind is likely to hold you back. Besides, who wants to spend the last precious seconds to count-down thinking about something else?

Work with your body, not your mind. When you want to delay ejaculation, stop doing whatever it is that's pushing you toward the inevitable. Hold totally still for a few seconds or even a few minutes. Or get up and change positions. Then slowly start again.

This man went on to say that coming so fast made him feel like less of a man because he thought everyone lasted at least 15 to 20 minutes. Let's put that one to rest right now. The average guy, having average sex in an average situation, lasts about 3 minutes. Is that slow, fast, or in between? Who knows? Remember, it's about satisfaction.

Nearly all men come quicker than they'd like on occasion. For the most part, though, it's more of an issue with young men without a lot of experience. Other factors also come into play. Men who have sex infrequently are more likely to come quickly than those who have it often. Nervousness can also make you a bit quick on the trigger. This is part of the reason that so many men come much more quickly with new partners. Studies suggest that premature ejaculation is less likely to occur when a man and woman know each other well, are comfortable with themselves, and are enjoying each other in a relaxed, no-rush setting.

We discuss techniques for managing premature ejaculation in quite a bit of detail in chapter 5. In brief, here are the main ones.

MASTER MASTURBATION. It's a great way to practice holding off because you control the timing, the intensity, and everything else. Practice working yourself up until you're almost ready to come, then back off. Try to do it at least two or three times before you let yourself go. At the same time, pay attention to the physical sensations that you experience as you move toward orgasm. The sooner you recognize the signs, the easier it will be to hold off when you're with a partner.

STOP AND GO. When you feel yourself reaching the point of orgasm during sex, stop moving entirely. Just lie there and let things calm down. Once the urge to ejaculate subsides, start moving again, but slowly. Keep doing this for as long as you're able.

SQUEEZE TO STOP. When an orgasm feels imminent, stop moving and firmly squeeze your penis just below the head. Maintain the pressure until the urge to have an orgasm fades. Then go back to what you were doing, squeezing at intervals until you're ready to call it quits.

BREATHE DEEPLY. Pause to take a few slow, lung-filling breaths as you move toward orgasm. It will help curtail the need to come, while at the same time helping you maintain your erection.

COMMUNICATE WELL AND OFTEN. Tell your partner that you're about to come, and ask her to slow down or stop for a minute or two. She won't mind, especially if slowing down allows you both to enjoy the intimacy longer.

CHANGE POSITIONS. Some positions, such as man on top, are a lot more stimulating for men than others, such as lying side by side. When you're trying to get your orgasms under control, stick to positions that are a little less stimulating for you.

CREAM THE SENSATIONS. Available in pharmacies, desensitizing creams temporarily numb the penis and can give better control. Another option is to wear a condom or even two to reduce friction.

IMPROVE MUSCULAR CONTROL. Exercises called Kegels, which involve clenching the same muscle that you'd use to stop the flow of urine, are among the best ways to control ejaculation. We describe the whole Kegels program in chapter 5. Suffice it to say that strong pelvic, abdominal, and butt muscles allow you to get control over ejaculatory sensations before they push you over the brink.

BIT PLAYERS IN THE SEX SCENE

Premature ejaculation and difficulty getting or keeping erections are the main sexual problems men face, but there are quite a few others. They're not as common, but they can make sex just as unsatisfying if they aren't taken care of. Many of these problems are caused, in whole or part, by underlying medical problems, so be sure to see your doctor if any of the following apply to you.

▶ Anejaculation. It means that you're able to come, but no semen comes out. It usually occurs in men who have had prostate surgery or spinal cord injuries.

▶ Delayed ejaculation. As with premature ejaculation, there are no strict time limits to define what's delayed, though 30 to 40 minutes is probably about average. Suffice it to say that men with delayed ejaculation can take forever to come. They get frustrated, and their partners get sore. It's usually caused by psychological rather than physical factors.

▶ Ejaculatory impotence. Also known as inhibited male orgasm, it means a man can sustain an erection for a long time, but can't come inside a woman. He may, however, be able to come in other ways. Psychological factors are usually to blame.

▶ Peyronie's disease. It's a harmless, though sometimes painful, condition that occurs when fatty deposits form on tissues inside the penis. Because the deposits are quite hard, erections make a detour and deflect around them, causing the penis to curve to one side. You might be able to feel the deposits along the top of the shaft. Medications will sometimes break up the deposits. In severe cases, surgery may be needed.

▶ Priapism. Basically, it means you get very long-lasting erections. They last so long that the pressure of blood in the penis can cause excruciating pain. There can also be tissue damage due to impaired circulation. Priapism can be caused by injuries to the penis or by the use of drugs (such as papaverine or, less often, Viagra) used to promote erections. Your doctor can give an injection to immediately release the erection. Be sure to get medical help; priapism can cause permanent damage.

▶ Retrograde ejaculation. It sometimes occurs after prostate surgery. The ejaculate travels backward into the bladder rather than out of the end of the penis. It isn't harmful, but it can be a disconcerting experience—and may make a man sterile in some cases. Your doctor will probably advise you to ignore it, although there are drugs that can send the ejaculate in the proper direction.

OBJECTIVE HELP

More than a few sex therapists in the swinging '70s took a hands-on approach to resolving lovemaking laments. These days (sorry), the approach is predictably a leather couch, a notepad, and professional attire.

But some things never change. The average man would rather volunteer for a lifetime of toilet cleaning than write a hefty check to slink into a therapist's office and discuss his sex life. That's unfortunate because nearly all of the sexual problems that men encounter, including those caused in part by physical factors, can be greatly improved with counseling. For example, some studies suggest that up to 98 percent of men who experience premature ejaculation have partial or total success after working with a therapist.

Sex, and sex problems in particular, is hard to talk about. The advantage of seeing a therapist is that you can talk to someone who knows the issues as well as the solutions and who isn't personally vested in your life. Therapy provides a neutral environment, in other words— a place to focus on solutions rather than passing around the blame.

Sex therapy incorporates elements of psychotherapy, behavior modification, and plain old marriage counseling. It takes a wide-angle view of your background and personality before zeroing in on the details of the problems that brought you through the door. If anything, sex therapy tends to deemphasize the sexual side of things until both you and the therapist have a better handle on what makes you tick.

None of us lives in a sexual vacuum. Your relationships, current as well as past, probably have more to do with your sexual happiness than the machinery involved. Even if it's your sexual issues that steered you into counseling, you may find that your partner has some issues of her own, including issues she never mentioned to you. Studies suggest that up to a third of clients in sex therapy have partners with their own sexual issues. Therapy gives you both a chance to clear the air and, more important, decide what to do next.

You might spend some time talking about your relationships, the dog you used to love, and the miserable time you had in high school. But you'll get a lot of very specific suggestions for dealing with the issues at hand: Exercises to improve ejaculatory control, for example, or mental techniques for overcoming erection problems. Therapists have seen, or at least talked about, just about everything. Nothing is off-limits. You might be embarrassed by the specificity of the discussions, but your therapist won't be.

One important caveat: Few states license sex therapists, so it's up to you to check out their credentials. In general, you want a therapist who has an advanced degree—a doctorate in psychology, for example, or a master's in social work. Quite a few good therapists without advanced degrees work in conjunction with psychologists or doctors.

They have excellent training and will probably be less expensive than a psychologist or psychiatrist specializing in sexual issues. The American Association of Sex Educators, Counselors, and Therapists offers a practitioner locator on their Web site, www.aasect.org.

THE ISSUE OF SIZE

Sigmund Freud insisted that the sex most preoccupied with penises was the one without them. Let's not kid ourselves.

A lot of men, especially when they're young, are almost obsessed with the size of their penises. They desperately want to know that they're well hung, or at least hung well enough. The problem is that few of us really know what other men look like. The occasional glance in a locker room doesn't tell much, and standing in a circle comparing lengths doesn't exactly fall within culturally acceptable bounds.

Most of us grow up and make peace with the flesh we were born with, but some men are so worried about size that they get painfully self-conscious. They're so self-conscious in some cases that they have trouble getting erections when someone is watching—and, they fear, judging.

It might help if they knew that the average penis is roughly between 5 and 7 inches long when erect. It doesn't matter how big your thumbs or nose are, either. A small man can easily have a larger than average penis, just as a big guy can have a relatively small one.

"I think the average man wishes he were better endowed," a 40-year-old account executive told us. *"We tend to equate penis size with virility and appeal as a lover. Though I'm well within the average range, I would like to have a longer, thicker member, just because I think it's more manly."*

Here's a guy who measures just fine. Most women would be perfectly satisfied with what he brings to bed. But he still dreams of more. That's unfortunate because this guy, and millions of other

American men, is putting himself through the emotional wringer for something that's entirely normal, that women are pleased with, and that he can't control.

No one can stop you from dreaming similar dreams. No matter how much intelligence and common sense you bring to the issue, you may find yourself wondering about all of the exercises, stretches, and surgical techniques that have been developed, with varying degrees of legitimacy, to increase the size of the penis. Yes, it is possible to do it, and it's worth discussing some of these techniques so you'll know what's out there. But unless you're unusually small—so small that normal intercourse is a problem—you'd be a lot better off praising nature for what you have. The women you're with don't care, so why should you?

STRETCH FOR MORE?

Stretching and squeezing penises to increase their length has a long history. In China and the Middle East, such techniques are still practiced today. Prepubescent Arabic boys, for example, practice the Jelq "milking" technique to shape their penises into respectably sized maturity. Increasing circulation through the tissues could theoretically make the penis longer and thicker when erect. Whether it actually does this, though, hasn't been well studied—and the gain, if any, is likely to be measured in fractions of an inch. This series of exercises based on this traditional practice *might* increase penis size if done daily for at least 6 months.

WARM IT UP. Soak a washcloth in warm water, wring it out, and wrap it around your penis for 5 to 10 minutes to increase bloodflow. Ideally, you should be erect or semi-erect at the time.

PINCH AND STRETCH. After your penis is warm, give yourself a genital massage. Pinch and stretch different parts of the scrotal sac for 5 seconds each.

MASSAGE EACH TESTICLE. Cup your testicles in your left hand. Use your right hand to gently massage them for 30 seconds.

Then cup them in your right hand and massage with the left. Take an extra minute to massage, pull, and knead the scrotum while holding one testicle in each hand.

GREASE IT UP. Rub some lotion or massage oil onto the shaft of your penis. Circle your thumb and forefinger around the base of the shaft. Squeeze firmly for 5 seconds, then release. Repeat the squeeze, moving slowly up the shaft.

REAPPLY LUBRICATION IF NECESSARY. Form a ring with your thumb and forefinger and slide it slowly and smoothly up the shaft toward the tip. As you get close to the top, use your other hand to start the process again from the bottom. Continue this double stroking for up to 10 minutes.

Will massaging and stretching the penis really increase its size? No one knows for sure. The whole process will certainly feel good, though, and if you enjoy it, well, keep it up.

SIZE FOR SALE

Doctors use a variety of stretching devices after penis surgery to prevent scar tissue from accumulating, but they're not recommended for at-home use. Nor are they designed to increase penis size.

There are products, however, that may increase size incrementally. Penis pumps are a variation on the age-old technique of suspending a weight from the penis in order to lengthen it—a technique that's painful and potentially dangerous. The pumps are safer and probably more effective, at least in the short run.

Originally created for men with diabetes, who often have vascular problems that inhibit erections, the pumps force blood into the penis, engorging and stretching the tissues. In addition, the suspensory ligament, which holds an erection upright, is pulled outward by the vacuum and *may* get somewhat longer over time.

The pumps consist of a plastic tube 8 or so inches long and 3 inches wide, a hand or electric pump (hand models are recommended for novices), and a flexible ring that secures around the base of the penis to prevent blood from escaping. You put your penis into the tube and pump out the air. Pressure from the vacuum causes blood to gather in your penis. Once you're hard, apply the ring to the base of the penis to trap the blood.

The pumped-up penis usually stays that way for about an hour, even after the ring is removed. (Always remove the ring within 30 minutes to restore normal blood circulation and prevent injury.) Optimists claim that using the pumps several times a week might result in a permanent increase in penis size, but it's unlikely that this actually occurs. You will get bigger, but only temporarily.

Quality pumps average about $150. You can find them on the Internet on sites such as www.MyPleasure.com and www.Xandria.com.

A KINDER CUT?

A very, very small percentage of men have penises that are too small for adequate intercourse. They can gain an inch or more with an experimental surgical procedure called phalloplasty, which basically rearranges fatty tissues and ligaments in the penis to add length as well as girth.

The experts we talked to agreed that it's insane for a man with a more or less normal size penis to even contemplate having the surgery—and unethical for surgeons to perform it except in cases when lengthening the penis will have profound effects on a man's health or well-being. An example might be a man whose penis is only an inch or two long when erect.

However, the high cost of this essentially cosmetic procedure, about $4,000, guarantees that surgeons in search of a buck will gladly perform it—and more than a few men with *normal* penises have been eager to have it.

Regardless of the pros and cons, here's what the surgery involves.

LENGTHENING PROCEDURES. The suspensory ligament, which anchors the penis to the body and holds it up during erections, extends a couple of inches under the skin. Pulling the ends outward slightly adds length to the penis—usually between 1 and 1½ inches. Men who have the procedure usually use a medical stretching device for several months after surgery to allow the penis to heal at its maximum length.

The downsides: Scar tissue that forms after surgery could pull the ligament back to its original position, in which case you're out of pocket and out of luck. The procedure doesn't always deliver the promised results. The penis might be longer when flaccid but gain nothing when erect.

Low libido accounts for roughly half of all admissions to sex therapy clinics.

GIRTH PROCEDURES. To the extent that women care about size at all, they usually prefer a man who's thick to one who's long—and surgery can make your penis somewhat thicker. Surgeons use several techniques. The oldest and possibly the least effective, called lipotransfer, involves liposuctioning fat from the thighs and buttocks and injecting it under the skin of the penis. Some of the fat is reabsorbed into the body, so the gains aren't as impressive as they initially seem.

Another technique, dermal fat grafts, involves taking a strip (rather than liposuctioned bits) of fat from the buttocks and tucking it into the penis like a strip of bacon. In live tissue transfer, the third procedure, fat from the pubic area is loosened at one end and flipped over into the shaft of the penis. Since the fat is still attached to the pubic area at one end, it maintains its original blood supply and presumably stays intact longer.

INDEX